Atlas of Liver Biopsies

Atlas of Liver Biopsies

Atlas of Liver Biopsies
1st edition

Copyright © 1979 Munksgaard, Copenhagen

Cover by Michael Clante.

Printed in Denmark by Johnsen+Johnsen, Copenhagen.

ISBN 87-16-2187-8

Distributed in North and South America by
J. B. Lippincott Company.

ISBN 0-397-58252-8

Atlas of Liver Biopsies

Hemming Poulsen & Per Christoffersen

MUNKSGAARD

North and South America:
J. B. LIPPINCOTT COMPANY

Acknowledgments

Our thanks are due to the many colleagues, pathologists as well as clinicians, with whom we have cooperated both scientifically and in the daily routine. We want especially to thank members of the following groups of which both or one of us are members: The Copenhagen Study Groups for Liver Diseases (CSL), The Copenhagen Hepatitis Acuta Programme (CHAP) and The European Liver Study Group.

Last, but not least, our sincere thanks are due to professor Peter Scheuer and to Hans Lyon, M.D., who have both shown great kindness in offering advice with regard to the English language.

Preface

In this atlas we have in a systematic fashion classified, described, and illustrated the most important of the numerous, individual, light microscopical lesions which are known to occur in liver tissue as a result of different physiological states and diseases. The function of the book is therefore to present the "building blocks" which form part of the morphological pictures of such conditions.

The atlas is intended mainly for general pathologists and for pathologists in training as a help in their diagnostic work, and for clinicians who seek information about liver biopsy diagnostics. The basis is the experience won by the authors during routine and scientific work with more than 11,000 liver biopsies during the past 12 years. As most of our biopsy material consists of liver biopsies from adults, the book only peripherally deals with childhood liver pathology.

Chapter I in connection with the technical appendix concerns our experience in the handling of liver biopsies.

Chapter II, the main chapter, is divided into sections which each deal with a separate morphological alteration or lesion. The sections follow a fairly uniform pattern, beginning with a morphological description supported by accompanying illustrations. This is followed by paragraphs concerning diagnosis and differential diagnostic problems. Finally a description is given of the conditions in which the particular morphological change has been seen and its significance is discussed. Parts of the text are to some degree repetitive because we want to keep references to other pages in the book at a minimum.

Chapter III, concerning the combination of the individual morphological changes, demonstrates how the so-called constant and inconstant features may lead not only to a diagnosis but also often give a clue to activity and prognosis. This chapter deals with only a few of the more important liver disorders; thus this book is not an alternative but a complement to the existing text books on liver pathology.

The nomenclature is, as far as possible, in accordance with "Diseases of the liver and biliary tract. Standardization of nomenclature, diagnostic criteria and diagnostic methodology," Fogarthy International Center Proceedings No. 22, 1976, and "The morphology of cirrhosis: definition, nomenclature, and classification," *Bulletin of the World Health Organization 55,* 521–540, 1977.

Contents

Chapter I

Processing of the Liver Biopsy

Introduction

Liver biopsy has for decades played an important role in the investigation of liver diseases. With modern techniques it is a safe procedure, and it is regularly used in all centers where liver diseases are studied. Its use, together with clinical and functional studies, has added greatly to our knowledge of a wide range of diseases of the liver, and it provides tissue which in addition to routine diagnostic work is also suitable for histochemical, immunological, and electron microscopic investigations which can often not be carried out successfully on autopsy material.

Lightmicroscopic evaluation of a liver biopsy specimen may confirm or exclude a possible clinical diagnosis, reveal an unexpected, sometimes significant disease, or be non-contributory or even misleading[1, 21]. In many cases an assessment of activity and extent as well as prognosis of the liver disease can be given[2], but for most disorders of the liver final diagnosis is the result of an overall assessment of exhaustive clinical, biochemical, physiological, immunological, radiological and histological investigations.

The use of liver biopsies is not restricted to patients with liver diseases. It also forms part of the investigation of a number of systemic and non-hepatic disorders including carcinomatosis, leukemias, lymphomas, pyrexia of unknown origin and granulomatous diseases.

The method has its limitations. The sample of tissue obtained is small, but despite the earlier doubts of many pathologists it proves adequate in a majority of cases. Its value, however, depends to a considerable extent on the histological processing and the interpretation of the biopsy specimen obtained. It is therefore of the utmost importance that both procedures are carried out optimally. One of the biggest problems in the interpretation of liver biopsies is sampling error. An average liver biopsy comprises one fifty-thousandth to one hundred-thousandth of the whole liver, and many of its diseases, not only focal processes such as granulomas and tumors, but also cirrhosis and chronic hepatitis, are more or less irregularly distributed. By being aware of these problems the interpreter cannot overcome them, but mistakes can be minimized.

Since the main stress in this atlas is put on the histological processing and the light microscopic interpretation of the liver biopsy, indications, contraindications, risk and complications as well as the technique of biopsy will not be discussed. For these topics the reader is referred to the relevant textbooks[9, 22].

Performance of Needle Biopsies

The first systematic attempt at needle biopsy of the liver appears to be that of Iversen & Roholm who in 1939 published their investigation of the histopathology of the liver in acute hepatitis on the basis of 160 percutaneous liver biopsies[12]. This paper stimulated the now widespread use of the method, and from this time onward a constantly increasing number of studies and reports has appeared in the literature.

Approach: Iversen & Roholm used the *percutaneous* route for performing the biopsy and this is still the usual method. The method is blind in that it does not to any great extent take focal lesions into consideration. The point of insertion is commonly intercostal, but may be subcostal.

In recent years advances in ultrasonic techniques have made it possible to locate focal lesions as small as 2 cm i diameter, and the performance of *percutaneous* needle liver biopsy in combination *with ultrasonic scanning* is found to be more accurate than the usual blind method in patients with focal lesions[16].

Needle biopsy under *peritoneoscopic control* makes it possible to remove tissue under direct vision and represents a useful diagnostic procedure in cases of macronodular (irregular) cirrhosis and focal lesions such as primary and secondary hepatic neoplasms. Biopsies performed through a peritoneoscope are often smaller and more fragmented than percutaneous specimens.

It must also be pointed out that even during *operation* a needle biopsy may be preferable to a small and mainly subcapsular surgical excision.

A recently introduced method, the so-called *transjugular* method, makes it possible to obtain liver tissue from patients with very low prothrombin time or with pronounced ascites[8, 20]. We have only limited experience with biopsies obtained by this route, but it is our impression that, although the specimens are on average smaller and more fragmented than those obtained by the percutaneous route, this method is a useful diagnostic procedure in selected patients.

Main types of biopsy needle: Many types of biopsy needle are available. The original cutting needle of Vim Silverman modified by Franklin is still popular in many places and is in many ways the best needle for biopsy of the cirrhotic liver. In our experience biopsy material obtained with this type of needle is usually marked by artefacts especially in the marginal areas, where the tissue is compressed and difficult to evaluate.

The trocar and cannula of Iversen & Roholm, though producing a large specimen, suffers from the disadvantage that it is a non-cutting instrument and therefore often results in distortion of the specimen.

More than 90 per cent of the biopsies we receive are performed with the technique and needle introduced by Menghini[15]. Most of the biopsies performed with this needle are 2 cm in length or more, often exceeding 3–4 cm and only exceptionally less than 1 cm. They are usually not fragmented and less marked by artefacts than is the case with biopsies removed with the other types of needle mentioned.

Performance of Surgical Biopsies

As mentioned previously a needle biopsy may in some cases be preferable to a biopsy taken with a knife, particularly if the specimen is small and mainly comprises subcapsular tissue. A necessary condition of an adequate surgical biopsy specimen is that it should be large – at least 10 x 10 x 10 mm – and that biopsy is performed from the anterior surface as far as possible from the hepatic margin[6].

A surgical or needle biopsy taken during operation or under peritoneoscopic control has the advantage that it can be performed from areas of the liver which are macroscopically found to be suitable. If it is large, a surgical biopsy has the additional advantage of comprising larger portal tracts than are normally found in needle biopsies; there is thus for instance a better chance of finding changes of the primary biliary cirrhosis type[5].

It is recommended that biopsy should be performed early during the operation since otherwise so-called surgical necrosis may obscure parenchymal detail and hamper diagnosis[6].

Handling of the Biopsy at the Bedside

Consistency of the liver: A record of the consistency of the liver and the naked eye appearance of the biopsy should be made at the time of the biopsy procedure. The liver is tough on biopsy in cirrhosis and in some patients with neoplasms, while in some examples of congenital hepatic fibrosis a biopsy may be unobtainable because of this factor.

Naked eye appearance: The liver biopsy is commonly fragmented in cirrhosis and sometimes in neoplasia; rarely normal liver tissue may also be fragmented. The combination of a tough liver and a fragmented biopsy is very suggestive of cirrhosis (Fig. 1).

The biopsy is green in cases with conspicuous cholestasis, irrespective of its etiology. In centrilobular cholestasis a regular pattern can often be seen with the naked eye (Fig. 2). The tissue is black in the Dubin-Johnson syndrome and dark brown in severe siderosis. In passive congestion a dark red color, often with alternating light and dark areas, is characteristic. The specimen may be pale in fatty change, and when steatosis is severe the tissue floats on the fixative. It is often mottled or uniformly white in patients with neoplasia. Malignant melanoma may be black (Fig. 3), and in cirrhosis the color is sometimes seen to vary, with whitish, brownish, yellow or green areas.

If photographs are required they should, if possible, be taken before the specimen is placed in the fixative, since the latter rapidly alters the color and the general appearance of the fresh specimen.

Careful attention to the gross appearances may thus be of diagnostic value. It is also important for assessing whether the final histological sections are representative of the whole material.

Initial treatment: In most cases the whole biopsy cylinder is treated for embedding in paraffin, but as several other techniques are available, it is necessary to make a decision before the performance of the biopsy whether any of these are to be used. Once the specimen has been placed into a fixative such as formalin the amount of information one can get from electron microscopy, histochemical and immunological investigations or chemical analysis is limited.

For *routine light microcopy* the biopsy is removed from the needle with great care and placed in a relatively large volume of a suitable fixative. It is important that the specimen is placed in the fixative immediately (Fig. 5). We have found it of no advantage to allow the biopsy to adhere to paper, cardboard or special metal grids, and instead we use small cylinder glasses

in which the biopsy lies free in the fixative. For routine diagnostic work the specimen is best transported in the fixative. Since it is often of importance to know the fixation time, especially when histochemical procedures are to be used, the date and time of biopsy should be noted on the written requisition form which accompanies the biopsy from the clinical department to the laboratory.

Tissue for *electron microscopy* should be placed in the appropriate fixative and cut into small pieces less than 1 mm^3 in size immediately or at the most within 1 minute after the biopsy is removed. As the preparative stages are extremely critical, it is desirable that this should be done by someone experienced in electron microscopic techniques. The place of electron microscopy in routine diagnostic work remains limited at present, although its role in research is well established. There are only a few and uncommon diseases in which a diagnosis can be established by electron microscopy but not under the light microscope; no doubt the number of these will increase.

Frozen sections may be used for rapid diagnosis and for staining of fat. If a qualitative examination for porphyrins is to be made, part of the biopsy should be used for frozen sections or for preparing a smear onto a glass slide for the detection of red fluorescence[14]. When certain histochemical (e.g. enzyme) or immunological (e.g. Hb_cAg, HB_eAg) investigations are to be carried out, part of the biopsy must be stored at –70°C for later frozen sections[10, 19].

The amount of tissue necessary for *chemical analysis* (for instance of glycogen, lipids, DNA and metals) and its handling varies according to the substance to be investigated and textbooks dealing with these problems must be consulted. In many cases the use of standard instruments and standard liquids may cause sufficient contamination to upset the results.

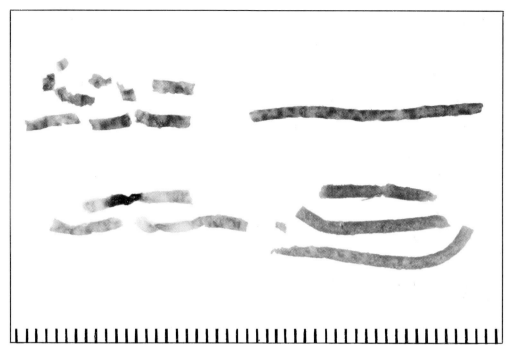

Figures 1–4: 1: Fragmented biopsy from a cirrhotic liver. 2: Biopsy from a case of acute viral hepatitis with conspicuous cholestasis. 3: Biopsy with metastases from malignant melanoma. 4: Five cm long biopsy cut into 3 pieces. The scale indicates mm.

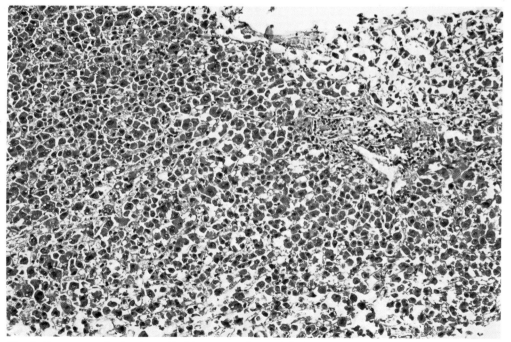

Fig. 5: From a poorly fixed needle biopsy stored overnight in 0.9 per cent watery sodium chloride. Re-biopsy a few days later revealed typical acute viral hepatitis (H & E x 110).

Handling of the Biopsy in the Laboratory

Procedures for routine light microscopy: Fixation. As the fixative of choice we have used 3.6 per cent neutral, buffered formaldehyde solution (10 per cent formalin)[13, 17]. It is the most commonly used, and all pathologists are familiar with the relatively minor artefacts produced in tissues fixed in this way. Another important advantage is that although the formaldehyde is bound chemically to the tissue, this binding is to some extent reversible, so that many histochemical procedures can be carried out after fixation.

There are also some disadvantages which can, however, be reduced considerably by fixing for only a short time (approximately 1 hour). One disadvantage is that glycogen disappears in a partly unpredictable manner from the tissue, and another is that formaldehyde-fixed material is not optimal for immunohistochemical investigations.

Bouin's solution, containing formaldehyde, picric acid and acetic acid, gives a very satisfactory light microscopic picture and is well suited for immunohistochemistry, whereas it is unfitted for most histochemical investigations, especially for copper and nucleic acids[13, 17].

Lillie's AAF solution, comprising ethanol, acetic acid and formaldehyde, has the same general properties as Bouin's solution. Lillie's fluid is particularly suited for demonstration of mucins[13, 17].

Dehydration. We use short dehydration of 1½ hour (see technical appendix). This gives an appearance which is less marked by artefacts than when using longer times, and the procedure gives good results in particular at the cytological level.

Embedding. For routine use embedding in paraffin ("paraplast") is preferable, and here also it is important to use a procedure as short as possible in order to keep artefacts at a minimum (see technical appendix). It is essential that during the processing the melting point of the paraffin (56–60°C) should be reached but not exceeded.

It is also essential that the tissue be placed into the paraffin in such a way that all of it is on the same horizontal plane. This is nearly impossible with long unbroken biopsies, and such biopsies should therefore be cut into pieces of 1–1½ cm each (Fig. 4).

In smaller series we have used other embedding materials for routine work. Epon embedded tissue can be cut in 1 or 2 μm sections. The process results in better preservation of both cellular and structural detail. The thinner sections provide clearer delineation of inflammatory infiltrates, cellular changes, and intracellular deposits. This method will probably be a valuable alternative to conventional paraffin embedding[4].

Sectioning. For routine work we have found that sections 5 μm thick are most suitable. When the sections are considerably thicker many details are obscured, and when sections are cut thinner it is often difficult or impossible to evaluate the architecture of the tissue.

It is our experience that a large number of consecutive sections are an advantage, and we use 54 numbered sections (Fig. 6) from a serial microtome. It is usually possible to produce 150–180 serial sections from a conventional needle biopsy, and 54 sections will thus leave sufficient tissue for further investigations. The large number of sections is used because our experience has shown that this increases the possibility of finding focal changes such as granulomas. Furthermore the numbering of consecutive sections enhances the understanding of the third dimension with demonstration of, for instance, the extent of segmental bile duct lesions.

Staining. The choice of routine stains varies according to the preferences of the interpreter, but H & E and staining for reticulin and collagen fibers have been found indispensable. In addition it is usually very useful to perform PAS, PAS after diastase, orcein staining and staining for iron, and it is recommended that these procedures should be carried out on all biopsies.

For the demonstration of collagen fibers (Fig. 7) we prefer the van Gieson stain because it is much easier to differentiate the collagen fibers by this method than in Azan or trichrome stains. A disadvantage is that the red color gradually fades and may finally disappear completely.

Sections stained for reticulin fibers are superior

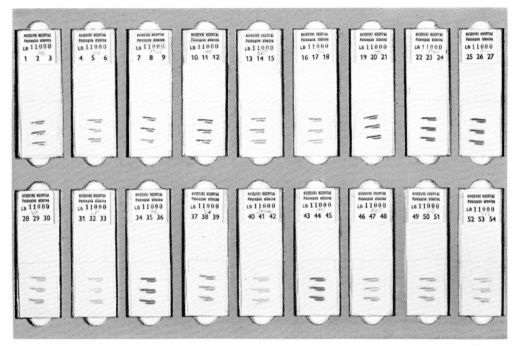

Fig. 6: Tray with 54 numbered, consecutive sections cut on a serial microtome. For the different stainings see Technical Appendix.

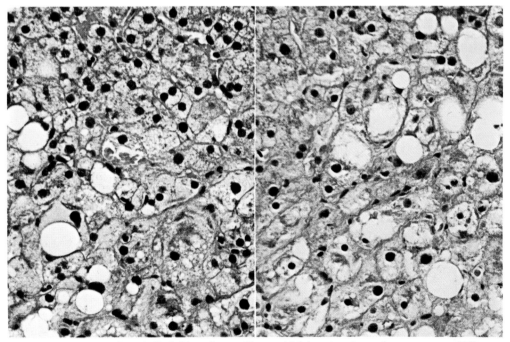

Fig. 7: Comparison of H & E (left) and van Gieson (right) stains from the same area (different sections). Note the ease with which collagen fibers are recognized in the latter (Needle biopsy x 270).

for the evaluation of architecture, whether the lobular architecture is preserved or nodule formation has taken place. These sections are in addition of value in the assessment of the limiting membrane and the liver cell plates, and in particular they are well suited for the demonstration of collapse of parts of the parenchyma (Fig. 8 and 9). By comparing with sections stained for collagen fibers it is possible to distinguish between collapsed areas and true fibrous septa as well as transitional forms.

PAS after diastase is particularly good for demonstration of some intracytoplasmic globules in the liver cells and ceroid, even in small amounts, in Kuppfer cells. Orcein staining is mainly used for differentiation between different types of so-called ground glass hepatocytes, but it is also of importance in screening for copper – containing granules in hepatocytes. When orcein – positive granules are present, special stains for copper should be applied.

Many laboratories prefer other stains than orcein for the demonstration of $HB_S Ag$ – positive ground glass hepatocytes, for example Gomori's aldehyde fuchsin. This is mainly due to the great variation in the staining properties of orcein from different sources. A reliable orcein staining procedure is given in the technical appendix.

Other stains which we regularly use include methyl green pyronin for nucleic acids (mainly for the demonstration of plasma cells in dense infiltrates of mononuclear cells), rubeanic acid (for copper) and methyl violet and Congo red (mainly for the demonstration of amyloid). Our staining procedures for light microscopy are given in the appendix.

Procedures for electron microscopy: The material is fixed in cold 2.5% glutaraldehyde and 2% paraformaldehyde in phosphate buffer, postfixed in 1% osmium tetroxide buffered with phosphate, dehydrated in ethanol, and embedded in Epon.

Procedures for frozen sections and chemical analysis: See page 12.

Examination of the Biopsy under the Light Microscope

It is of great value to have a formal procedure for the evaluation of the biopsy. Chapter II of this atlas is laid out in the manner which we have found to give the most valuable interpretation. A recommended way of achieving this is by filling in a form on which all lesions which should be searched for are listed (see contents of chapter II, p. 8).

Polarizing microscopy is useful for the demonstration of amyloid, malarial and schistosomal pigments, protoporphyrins and talc, and *ultra-violet microscopy* for the demonstration of porphyrins, vitamin A and lipofuscin.

When the light microscopic analysis is finished and conclusions have been drawn on the basis of morphological appearances, a final conclusion should be made taking clinical, biochemical, physiological, radiological and other results into account. It is of great value to come to a purely morphological conclusion before seeing the clinical data, since it is very difficult to be completely objective when such information is known.

Adequacy of the Biopsy

Biopsies obtained by needle puncture have been criticized as being insufficient as they represent only a small part of the whole organ. Furthermore, morphological changes including disturbances of the architecture are common in the subcapsular 3–4 mm in an otherwise normal liver, and the amount of tissue for diagnosis is therefore additionally reduced.

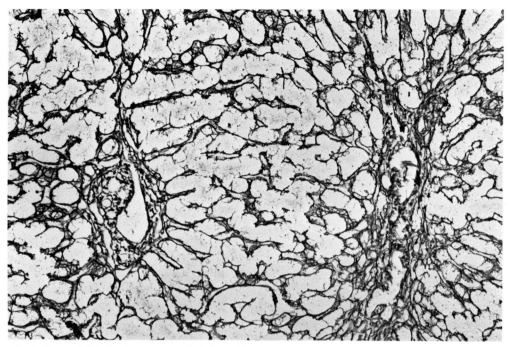

Fig. 8: Part of lobule from acute viral hepatitis with collapse of the reticulin framework around the central vein (right). A portal tract is seen in the left half of the picture (Needle biopsy, reticulin x 270).

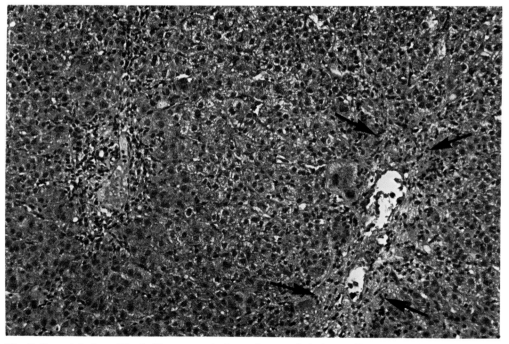

Fig. 9: Same lobule as Fig. 8. The arrows indicate the centrilobular confluent necrosis corresponding to the reticulin collapse. No new collagen was found with van Gieson stain (Needle biopsy, H & E x 270).

The adequacy of the biopsy depends not only on its size but is also related to the nature of the disease being investigated. If the disease involves the liver diffusely, as in viral hepatitis, it is obviously more likely to be revealed in a small biopsy than if the disease is focally distributed. Thus on an autopsy series diagnoses made on tissue taken from the liver with a biopsy needle were compared with diagnoses made on orthodox histological sections[7]. In several different diffuse conditions the correct diagnosis was made in 100 to 63 per cent of cases. In focal conditions the results again varied with the nature of the condition from 85 to 31 per cent. In a similar study in cirrhosis[3] it was found that when the parenchymal nodules are small, they are nearly always easy to recognize even in small fragmented biopsies, whereas large nodules may sometimes be difficult to identify, even in large biopsies, when they contain areas with preserved or partly preserved lobular architecture.

In an investigation of the reproducibility of diagnosis in relation to the size of the liver biopsy[11] it was shown that a diagnosis of viral hepatitis can be made with confidence on the appearance of only a few lobules (i.e. a biopsy of about 5 mm is sufficiently large). The diagnosis of large duct obstruction, however, requires many portal tracts[18] and a biopsy not less than 15 mm long, and the diagnosis of cirrhosis of macronodular type often requires a biopsy of more than 20–25 mm.

References

1. *Baggenstoss, A. H.:* Interpretation of liver biopsy without clinical data. The Journal-Lancet *82:* 234, 1962.

2. *Bianchi, L., De Groote, J., Desmet, V. J., Gedigk, P., Korb, G., Popper, H., Poulsen, H., Scheuer, P. J., Schmid, M., Thaler, H. & Wepler, W.:* Morphological criteria in viral hepatitis. Lancet *i:* 333, 1971.

3. *Braunstein, H.:* Needle biopsy of the liver in cirrhosis. Arch. Path. *62:* 87, 1956.

4. *Chi, E. Y. & Schmuckler, E. A.:* A rapid method for processing liver biopsy specimens for 2 μ sectioning. Arch. Pathol. Lab. Med. *100:* 457, 1976.

5. *Christoffersen, P., Poulsen, H. & Scheuer, P. J.:* Abnormal bile duct epithelium in chronic aggressive hepatitis and primary biliary cirrhosis. Human Pathol. *3:* 227, 1972.

6. *Christoffersen, P., Poulsen, H. & Skeie, E.:* Focal liver cell necrosis accompained by infiltration of granulocytes arising during operation. Acta Hepato-Splenologica (Stuttgart) *17:* 240, 1970.

7. *Christoffersen, P. & Povlsen, C. P.:* The adequacy of liver biopsy. A post mortem study comparing conventional histological sections with needle biopsies (not published results).

8. *Conn, H.:* Liver biopsy in extrahepatic biliary obstruction and in other "contraindicated" disorders. Gastroenterology *68:* 817, 1975.

9. *Edmondson, H. A. & Schiff, L.:* Needle biopsy of the liver. In: Schiff, L. (ed): Diseases of the liver, 4th, ed. Philadelphia: Lippincott, 247, 1975.

10. *Hopf, U., Meyer Zum Buchenfelde, K. H. & Freudenberg, J.:* Liver-specific antigens of different species. II Localization of a membrane antigen at cell surface of isolated hepatocytes. Clin. Exp. Immunol. *16:* 117, 1974.

11. *Hølund, B., Poulsen, H. & Schlichting, P.:* Reproducibility of liver biopsy diagnosis in relation to the size of the specimen (not published).

12. *Iversen, P. & Roholm, K.:* On aspiration biopsy of the liver, with remarks on its diagnostic significance. Acta med. scand. *102:* 1, 1939.

13. *Lillie, R. D. & Fullner, H. M.:* Histopathologic Technic and Practical Histochemistry, 4th. ed. New York: McGraw-Hill Book Compagny, 25, 1976.

14. *Lundvall, O. & Enerbäck, L.:* Hepatic fluorescence in porphyria cutanea tarda studied in fine needle biopsy smears. J. Clin. Path. *22:* 704, 1969.

15. *Menghini, G.:* One second needle biopsy of the liver. Gastroenterology 35, 190, 1958.

16. *Nørby Rasmussen, S., Holm, H. H., Kristensen, J. Kvist & Barlebo, H.:* Ultrasonically-guided liver biopsy. Brit.Med. J. *2:* 502, 1972.

17. *Pearse, A. G. E.:* Histochemistry. Theoretical and Applied, 3rd. ed.: Edingburgh & London: Churchill Livingstone, 70, 1968.

18. *Poulsen, H. & Christoffersen, P.:* Histological changes in liver biopsies from patients with surgical bile duct disorders. Acta path. microbiol. scand. Section A. *78:* 571, 1970.

19. *Raia, S. & Scheuer, P. J.:* Method for obtaining both frozen and paraffin sections from the same liver biopsy. J. Clin. Path. *21:* 413, 1968.

20. *Rösch, J., Lakin. P. G., Antonovic, R. & Dotter, C. T.:* Transjugular approach to liver biopsy and transhepatic cholangiography. N. Eng. J. Med. *289:* 227, 1973.

21. *Shorter, R. G.:* Liver biopsy. An atlas of histologic appearances. Oxford: Pergamon Press. 1961.

22. *Thaler, H.:* Leberbiopsie. Ein klinisches Atlas der Histopathologie. Berlin: Springer-Verlag. 13, 1969.

General Reading

Lillie, R. D. & Fullner, H. M.: Histopathologic Technic and Practical Histochemistry, 4th. ed. New York: Mc Graw-Hill Book Company, 1976.

Pearse, A. G. E.: Histochemistry. Theoretical and Applied, 3rd. ed. Edinburgh & London: Churchill Livingstone. 1968.

Schiff, L.: Diseases of the liver, 4th. ed. Philadelphia: Lippincott, 1975.

Sherlock, S.: Diseases of the liver and biliary system, 4th. ed., Oxford: Blackwell Scientific 1971.

Thaler, H.: Leberbiopsie, Berlin: Springer-Verlag 1969.

Chapter II

Individual
Morphological Features

Normal

Morphology: A liver lobule is decribed as a polygonal, prismatic formation constituting a mass of liver parenchyma which has in its center a central vein, and which is demarcated by planes connecting the adjacent portal tracts (Fig. 10) [118, 125, 220]. Under normal conditions one can demonstrate a radial arrangement of liver cell plates. The plates are one cell thick and on either side exposed to hepatic sinusoids which converge toward the smallest hepatic veins (central veins)[241]. Each central vein collects part of the blood from 3 to 4 or more portal tracts. As the term indicates, the central vein is regarded as the center of the lobule, whereas the portal tracts mark the periphery.

Rappaport, on the other hand, has put forward the concept of the functional unit, the acinus[299, 301] (Fig. 11). This is centered around an axis comprising terminal portal venules, hepatic arterioles, bile ducts, lymph vessels and nerves. The axis extends from a small triangular portal tract and is three dimensionally almost pear-shaped. An acinus has peripherally located central veins ("terminal hepatic veins"), and under the light microscope is composed of parts of adjoining "lobules". No capsular structures separate the acini.

Both the conventional lobules and the acinar concept are necessary tools for the understanding of the physiology of the normal liver and the morphogenesis of the different liver disorders. The two theories are complementary, and one does not exclude the other.

When, in the interpretation of a liver biopsy, one talks about normal or preserved lobular architecture, this means that it is possible to identify conventional lobules and acini, as well as portal tracts and central veins, throughout the whole biopsy. In addition one finds a distance between central veins and portal tracts of the magnitude of 400 to 700 μm, and a radial arrangement of liver cell plates around the central veins.

Morphological diagnosis: The histological recognition of preserved lobular architecture is easy as a rule. It is recommended to use low magnification of sections stained for reticulin fibers and sections stained with H & E.

If the biopsy is small and/or fragmented, it may be difficult or impossible to assess whether the lobular architecture is preserved or not. Tangentially cut portal tracts and central veins possibly combined with fibrosis may add further difficulties. Serial sections may in such cases be of some help, but repeat biopsy is often necessary.

Differential diagnosis: The most important differential diagnostic problem is macronodular cirrhosis, since parts of macronodules may show one-cell-thick plates with a certain degree of radial arrangement[43]. The irregular distribution of portal tracts and central veins, often together with areas of fibrosis, helps to exclude normal lobular architecture in nearly all cases.

A biopsy from a hepatocellular adenoma or well-differentiated hepatocellular carcinoma may similarly simulate preserved lobular architecture. In such cases the vessels are also irregularly distributed, and it is of differential diagnostic importance that adenomas contain no or only very few bile ducts[189].

Additional morphological findings: Liver tissue with preserved lobular architecture may be completely normal, but most of the portal and parenchymal changes described in this atlas may be found in livers with normal lobular architecture.

Occurrence and significance: In most series the majority of the biopsies show preserved lobular architecture. The most important diagnostic consideration is the exclusion of cirrhosis. In this context micronodular cirrhosis gives no problems[43]. Macronodular cirrhosis may, however, sometimes imitate preserved lobular architecture when only part of a large nodule is represented in the biopsy[137].

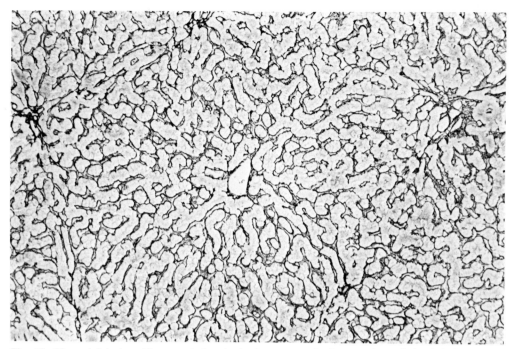

Fig. 10: Normal lobule with a central vein in its center. A demarcation of the lobule can be estimated by planes connecting adjacent portal tracts (Needle biopsy, reticulin x 110).

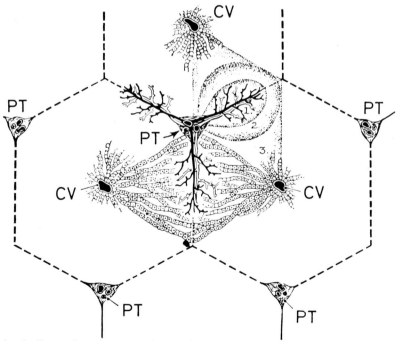

Fig. 11: A simple liver acinus is centered around an axis with a terminal hepatic arteriole, portal venule and bile duct. The acinus lies between two or more "central veins" (CV) and is subdivided into three circulatory zones like layers of an onion (PT: portal tracts).

Parenchymal nodules (cirrhosis)

Morphology: The most common form of destroyed lobular architecture is parenchymal or "regenerative" nodules. By a parenchymal nodule is meant a rounded portion of the parenchyma with smooth or sometimes slightly irregular outline. The nodules are composed of liver cells arranged in irregular, partly anastomosing plates[380]. Whereas the normal liver cell plate in adults and larger children is one cell thick and extends from a central vein to a portal tract[241], the plates in parenchymal nodules are usually of varying thickness and of different length. The plates in the nodules are as rule separated by sinusoids, but capillaries with dense collagen fibers in their walls can also be found. In other areas hyalinized connective tissue with only few vessels may be demonstrated[274].

Parenchymal nodules develop by sequestration of the original liver tissue by fibrous septa arising after extensive liver cell necrosis. Within each segment liver cells proliferate in order to try to replace the necrotic cells which have initiated the septum formation. This liver cell proliferation seems to be most pronounced in the vicinity of the septa, resulting in a rounding off of the segments. In this way the parenchymal nodules are formed[274].

If the sequestration affects all the lobules, the parenchyma is remodelled into small, relatively uniform nodules (Fig. 12) without central veins or portal tracts[309]. A considerable tendency to proliferation of the liver cells will eventually convert some of these small nodules to large nodules, possibly with a diameter of 2, 3 or more centimeters. In such nodules one usually finds one or more areas with localized dilatation of the sinusoids appearing very similar to central veins and possibly efferent in function[274].

If the sequestration is more irregularly distributed in the liver and does not involve every lobule, the parenchyma is tranformed into nodules, some of which are large and may contain areas with intact lobules with normal appearing portal tracts and central veins[309] (Fig. 13).

Morphological diagnosis: When the parenchymal nodules are small, they are virtually always easy to recognize even in small, fragmented biopsies[43].

On the other hand, large nodules may sometimes be difficult to identify when they comprise areas with preserved or partly preserved lobular architecture[43]. Use of serial sections with H & E and reticulin staining is indispensable in doubtful cases.

It is a well-known fact that a diagnosis of parenchymal nodules must not be made on subcapsular tissue since fibrosis in this area, for instance after acute hepatitis, may be associated with islands of liver cells very similar to nodules[266].

Differential diagnosis: Since the parenchymal nodules arise following sequestration of the lobules, all transitions between partly dissected lobules and fully developed nodules are seen. Assessment of the architecture may be especially difficult in the presence of severe steatosis. Similarly extensive confluent necrosis with portal-central bridging necrosis sometimes gives rise to architectural irregularities which may give a false impression of nodule formation in H & E-stained sections. Serial sections stained for reticulin usually allow a correct diagnosis to be made.

Additional morphological findings: All the histological changes found in cirrhosis may be present (chap. III).

Occurrence and significance: Widely distributed parenchymal nodules are nearly always accompanied by fibrosis, and the mutual presence of both is generally accepted as diagnostic of cirrhosis[7,274] (chap. III).

Parenchymal nodules may in addition be found in focal nodular hyperplasia and in nodular regenerative hyperplasia (see p. 26).

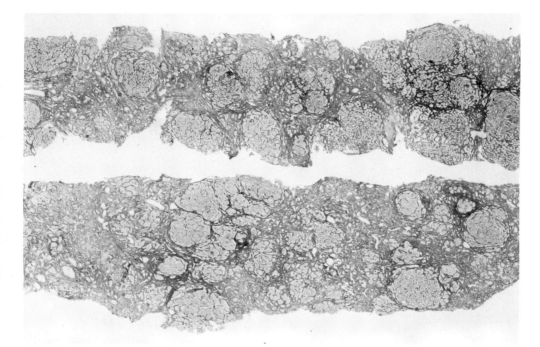

Fig. 12: Micronodular cirrhosis with small, relatively uniform parenchymal nodules surrounded by anastomosing septa of somewhat varying thickness. From a chronic alcoholic (Needle biopsy, reticulin x 30).

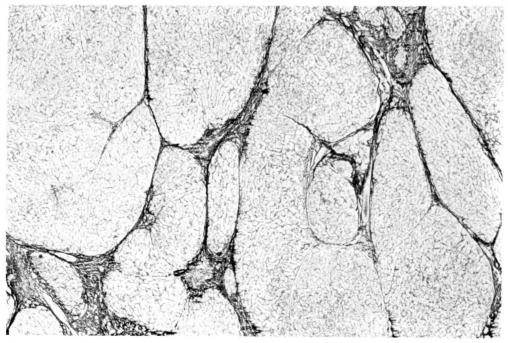

Fig. 13: Macronodular cirrhosis with nodules of varying size. The larger contain areas which simulate lobular architecture. The septa are more slender than in the micronodular cirrhosis. From a post-hepatitic cirrhosis, inactive for years (Surgical biopsy, reticulin x 30).

Parenchymal nodules (non-cirrhosis)

Morphology: The most common parenchymal nodules are widely distributed in the liver and associated with fibrosis. Two other types of parenchymal nodules are found in focal nodular hyperplasia and nodular regenerative hyperplasia.

Focal nodular hyperplasia (syn. "focal cirrhosis") is a focal change with parenchymal nodules and fibrosis. The lesion is most often solitary but two or more may be found. The size is usually 1 to 2 cm and the lesion is roughly globular with one or more central scars from which delicate septa radiate. Between the septa, nodules of varying size are present and in the septa there is bile duct proliferation, and a few inflammatory cells may be seen. The liver cells in the nodules usually contain more glycogen and fat than those of the surrounding parenchyma[111d, 189].

Nodular regenerative hyperplasia is a condition with widely distributed parenchymal nodules but no fibrosis (Fig. 14 & 15). The lobular architecture can still partly be recognized and the portal tracts and central veins identified. The nodules comprise the peripheral parts of the lobules corresponding to zone 1 and 2 of Rappaport's acinus, and centrilobularly (zone 3) there is sinusoidal dilatation and atrophy of the liver cell plates and in addition some liver cell necrosis. The plates in the parenchymal nodules run in different directions and are of varying thickness. The cells commonly exhibit a conspicuous variation in size and stainability. At low magnifications an impression of "reversed lobulation" is gained[360].

Morphological diagnosis: If a lesion of *focal nodular hyperplasia* should be sampled in a percutaneous biopsy it would probably be misdiagnosed as cirrhosis, but the chance of this happening is minimal, since the lesion is both rare and small. In surgical biopsies the diagnosis is usually easy.

In *nodular regenerative hyperplasia* the diagnosis is based on the parenchymal nodules representing periportal parts of the parenchyma and surrounded by atrophic liver cell plates, sinusoidal dilation, and absence of fibrosis[360].

Differential diagnosis: The differential diagnostic problem of *focal nodular hyperplasia* is cirrhosis. If a surgical biopsy is large and includes adjacent non-cirrhotic tissue, the chance of diagnostic error is minimal. If the biopsy is small, or is a needle biopsy, especially if adjacent non-cirrhotic tissue is missing, the misdiagnosis of cirrhosis can easily be made. The presence of central scarring is a helpful diagnostic sign. Focal nodular hyperplasia should also be distinguished from liver cell adenoma[189].

In H & E-stained sections *nodular regenerative hyperplasia* mainly resembles cirrhosis, in particular congestive or cardiac cirrhosis. The lack of dense collagen fibers around the nodules excludes the diagnosis of cirrhosis. A picture which architecturally may closely resemble nodular regenerative hyperplasia, though without sinusoidal dilatation, is seen in acute hepatitis with liver cell proliferation after confluent, centrilobular necrosis.

Additional morphological findings: In *focal nodular hyperplasia* the remaining parts of the liver are usually morphologically normal. *Nodular regenerative hyperplasia* is often accompanied by steatosis and centrilobular liver cell necrosis.

Occurrence and significance: *Focal nodular hyperplasia* is found in approximately 1 or 2 per cent of consecutive autopsy material. On gross inspection the lesion may look like a tumor – possibly a metastasis. It is probably a hamartoma, and benign[189, 360].

Nodular regenerative hyperplasia is relatively unusual in biopsy material. The congestion is most often caused by pronounced right-sided heart failure but may also be secondary to local lesions in relation to the inferior vena cava or hepatic vein such as thrombosis or tumor[86, 159]. Transition to cirrhosis may occur.

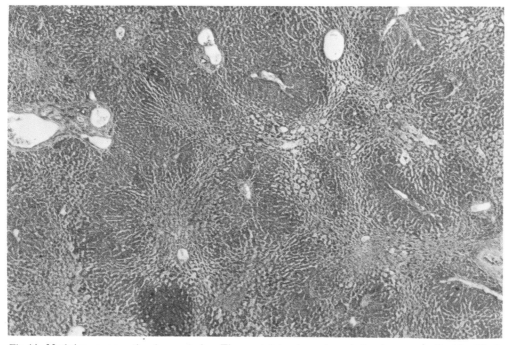

Fig. 14: Nodular regenerative hyperplasia. The portal tracts and central veins are easily identified. The changes give an impression of "reversed lobulation" around portal tracts. There is no fibrosis (Surgical biopsy, H & E x 30).

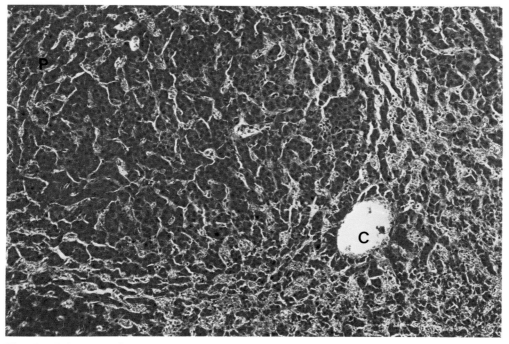

Fig. 15: Higher magnification with a nodule in the left side showing irregular plates of varying thickness. In the right side a central vein and sinusoidal dilatation with atrophy of the liver plates are seen (Same biopsy as above, H & E x 110).

Other abnormalities

Morphology: The lobular architecture of the liver can be altered in ways other than by formation of parenchymal nodules. The changes may be *focal,* comprising only few lobules including portal tracts, or *widespread* throughout the organ.

The *focal* changes may be present as irregularities of the liver cell plates, described on p. 72. Most often the focal changes are conditioned by inflammatory processes with scar formation, infarcts, or primary or secondary tumors. Smaller or larger areas of liver tissue are destroyed in relation to abscesses, gummata and granulomas. The adjacent parenchyma shows a partly concentric and more or less parallel arrangement of the liver cell plates as a result of compression (Fig. 16). There is in addition often infiltration by inflammatory cells. Another focal change is fibrosis (p. 154). Small stellate scars or rounded zones of newly formed collagen fibers may form after focal liver cell necrosis and lipogranulomas but is mainly seen after alcoholic hepatitis and in healing granulomatous diseases such as sarcoidosis. The number and size of the fibrous lesions depend on the underlying disease.

Liver cell carcinoma and adenoma in some cases imitate the normal lobular architecture, but in both tumors portal tracts and bile ducts are missing, and the trabeculae have an irregular extent and thickness. Furthermore, in liver cell carcinoma, cytological features of malignancy are demonstrable, and the adjacent liver tissue is usually cirrhotic.

Widespread changes in the liver arise as a consequence of extensive necrosis with centrilobular, periportal or bridging fibrosis (p. 158, 160 & 162). The disseminated fibrosis in congenital syphilis is interstitial[175]. Not only is the lobular architecture blurred, but true plates are missing and the liver cells are arranged in small groups or strands (Fig. 17). Widespread hepatic fibrosis is in addition seen following exposure to agents such as thorotrast[161, 384], inorganic arsenicals[244], methotrexate[250] and vinylchloride[284].

Morphological diagnosis: In order to diagnose the different forms of fibrosis adequately, it is necessary to have sections stained for collagen fibers. It is also necessary to use many sections in order to exclude the presence of cirrhosis.

Differential diagnosis: It may be difficult to distinguish changes following collapse of necrotic parenchyma from cirrhosis, especially when the necrosis is of bridging type. The use of serial sections and staining for both reticulin and collagen fibers usually makes the distinction possible.

Additional morphological findings: In the focal changes described one may, if the etiological factor is still active, see changes such as granulomas or tumor tissue. The same holds true for focal fibrosis and, for example, alcoholic hepatitis and lipogranulomas.

Bridging necrosis and bridging fibrosis are most common in chronic aggressive hepatitis and severe cases of acute hepatitis and, consequently, one finds parenchymal and portal changes typical of these diseases. The widespread fibrosis induced by thorotrast is accompanied by the typical pigment[161], and following vinyl chloride a characteristic proliferation of the sinusoidal lining cells is common[284].

Occurrence and significance: Small areas of fibrosis with irregularities of parts of the lobules are commonly found in alcoholics, and the lesion is often reversible. The same is the case for the usually slightly larger lesions following sarcoidosis. Many parenchymal granulomas may, however, form the basis for a portal-central bridging fibrosis and exceptionally also for cirrhosis.

Both cirrhosis and primary liver tumors may follow the described widespread changes which may develop after for instance acute and chronic hepatitis and after exposure to environmental agents such as thorotrast and vinyl chloride.

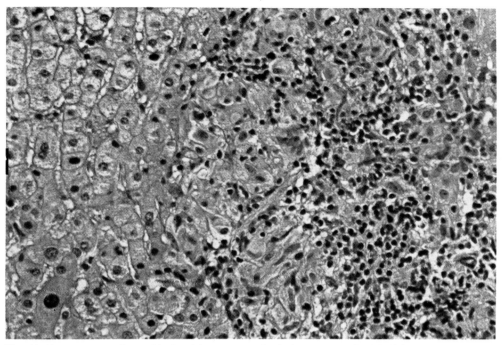

Fig. 16: From a case of sarcoidosis with an unusually high number of epithelioid cell granulomas both in portal tracts and parenchyma. Note the compressed parallel liver cell plates in the left side (Needle biopsy, H & E x 270).

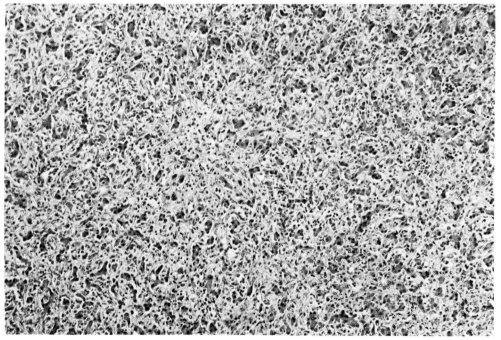

Fig. 17: Congenital syphilis. There is a widespread, interstitial, severe fibrosis separating many small groups of atrophic liver cells. No nodule formation (Autopsy, H & E x 30).

Normal

Morphology: Each portal tract includes an artery or arterioles, a branch of the portal vein, a bile duct or ducts, lymphatics and connective tissue (Fig. 18). The portal tract is delimited by a wall of liver cells called the limiting plate *(membrana limitans)*[11] and is more or less triangular on cross section. The tracts are, however, often rather long because of tangential cutting (Fig. 19). The larger portal tracts may show varying forms since the sections in many cases are taken through ramifications of the portal tree at different angles (Fig. 53). The portal tracts in a needle biopsy are usually all small, whereas in surgical biopsies larger tracts are also seen.

Bile ducts in small portal tracts are known as interlobular ducts[121, 358]. They are lined by cuboidal or low columnar epithelium. The ducts in the larger portal tracts are sometimes referred to as septal ducts[121, 358] and the epithelium is high columnar with basal nuclei. The connections between the ducts and the bile canaliculi of the parenchyma are the ductules and canals of Hering, the latter lined partly by cuboidal ductular cells and partly by liver cells[72, 358, 398]. Ductules are normally very scanty in a 4 to 5 µm section. The smallest portal tracts contain one bile duct, one portal vein branch and one arteriole[121]. The slightly larger tracts may contain one or two of each but the exact number varies. Medium sized portal tracts often contain two or three of each, but it is not unusual to find, for instance, two or three bile ducts and only one vein and one artery[156, 160]. The connective tissue in normal portal tracts consists of small, closely set bundles of collagen fibers and a network of reticulin, while there are only few fibroblasts. The picture is uniform throughout but a few lymphocytes and histiocytes may be found. Lymph vessels are normally inconspicuous. The same holds true for portal nerve branches, which can be demonstrated by special staining.

Morphological diagnosis: The histological recognition of normal portal tracts in a biopsy is easy as a rule. Low magnification is recommended of sections stained for collagen fibers and with H & E. Slight inflammation may, however, be overlooked, and it is therefore important in addition to use higher magnifications.

Differential diagnosis: The presence of portal tracts of varying sizes and more or less tangential sectioning may mimic portal or periportal fibrosis, or even slight bile duct proliferation. Some experience is necessary but if the portal tracts consists of uniform, mature connective tissue, are surrounded by normal limiting plates and the number and structure of bile ducts and vessels is estimated to be within normal limits, then a diagnosis of normal portal tracts can safely be made.

Additional morphological findings: If all the portal tracts in a biopsy are normal, other changes are usually absent. Normal portal tracts may, however, be seen in, for instance, "pure cholestasis" (p. 184) and in some cases of steatosis (p. 108), hemosiderosis (p. 120), and centrilobular sinusoidal dilation (p. 70).

Occurrence and significance: In most series only a minority of the biopsies show all portal tracts free of pathological changes. As mentioned above, this then often implies that the biopsy is normal.

The signifiance of normal portal tracts is mainly due to the fact that a considerable number of diagnoses can be excluded with a high degree of certainty, a prerequisite being that many (more than 10 to 15) portal tracts are represented in the biopsy. Examples of diagnoses excluded in this way are chronic aggressive hepatitis, cirrhosis, and large duct obstruction.

In this context it may be noted that in a number of biopsies with even severe conditions such as chronic aggressive hepatitis or large duct obstruction, one or a few normal portal tracts may be found.

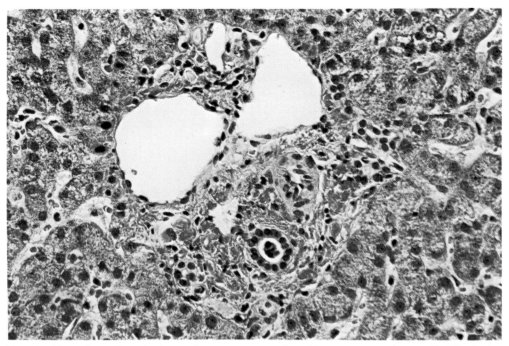

Fig. 18: Normal medium-sized portal tract, cross section. The space contains small bile ducts, ramifications of a portal vein branch and a centrally placed arteriole. The connective tissue contains thick bundles of collagen (Needle biopsy, van Gieson x 270).

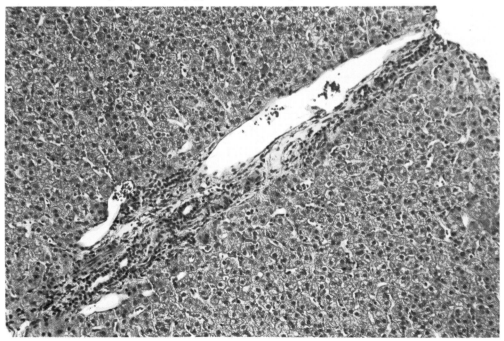

Fig. 19: Tangentially cut normal portal tract. The tract looks very long but contains the same elements as mentioned above (Needle biopsy, H & E x 110).

Predominance of neutrophils

Morphology: The majority of our liver biopsies show different degrees of inflammation in the portal tracts. The number of inflammatory cells varies from one tract to another but usually all portal tracts are involved. Neutrophils, eosinophils, lymphocytes, plasma cells and histiocytes are seen, and in some cases granulomas or lymphoid follicles. Occasionally only one cell type is present, but in most cases one cell type predominates.

Inflammation with predominance of neutrophils is nearly always localized in one of two ways. In the first and most common, the neutrophils are present mainly in the periphery of the portal tracts[67, 291], and in the second they are found mainly centrally in relation to the bile ducts[163, 373]. The number of neutrophils varies from very few to large numbers (Fig. 20 & 21), and in addition to neutrophils, lymphocytes and histiocytes are often to be found. On the other hand eosinophils and plasma cells are usually absent or scanty[67, 291].

Morphological diagnosis: Neutrophil granulocytes are easily identified in H & E-stained sections, and it is of importance to register both the degree of inflammation and the localization. Fig. 20 is an example of slight infiltration with neutrophils in the periphery of a portal tract and Fig. 21 an example of severe infiltration. Fig. 38, p. 51, shows neutrophils in relation to bile ducts.

Differential diagnosis: In the mildest degrees of infiltration with neutrophils the differential diagnostic problem is from a normal portal tract. In our experience even a few neutrophils are an expression of a pathological process.

Additional morphological findings: Inflammation with predominance of neutrophils in the periphery of the portal tracts is a very common finding in partial or complete obstruction of the larger bile ducts[67, 291]. A constant additional finding is a proliferation of smaller bile ducts with a marginal location and usually also edema.

Furthermore, centrilobular cholestasis is usually found, while other parenchymal changes are minor. In a long standing obstruction, liver cell necrosis may, however, develop in relation to the bile thrombi[67, 291].

Portal changes of the same type may also be found in biopsies with Mallory bodies, liver cell necrosis and neutrophils in the parenchyma[66] (alcoholic hepatitis, p. 92).

Predominance of neutrophils in portal tracts is occasionally seen together with lobular changes, as in acute hepatitis both of viral[265] and drug[187, 272] etiology (p. 172). On the other hand a few neutrophils can be found among other inflammatory cells in the portal tracts in approximately one half of the biopsies from acute hepatitis cases[265].

Neutrophils are often present in and around arterial walls in polyarteriitis nodosa. As a rule there is also infiltration by eosinophils, lymphocytes, plasma cells and histiocytes, and it is usually possible by serial sectioning to demonstrate fibrinoid precipitates and necrosis of the wall.

Occurrence and significance: The presence of many neutrophils in the periphery of the portal tracts, together with marginal bile duct proliferation and edema, speaks in favor of large duct obstruction[67, 291]. The lesion is, however, not pathognomonic, and similar changes may be found in some cases of acute hepatitis, particularly in cases with severe cholestasis[293].

The coexistence of portal changes with marginal bile duct proliferation, many neutrophils and edema and alcoholic hepatitis in the parenchyma, renders it probable that the patient has pancreatitis in addition to liver disease[333].

The presence of many neutrophils in the centrally situated portal bile ducts, especially when seen together with necrosis of the epithelium, is a good indication of bacterial infection. Scanty neutrophils either in the original bile duct or in the proliferating ducts in the margins of the tracts are a common finding in large duct obstruction and are not diagnostic for an ascending cholangitis[327f].

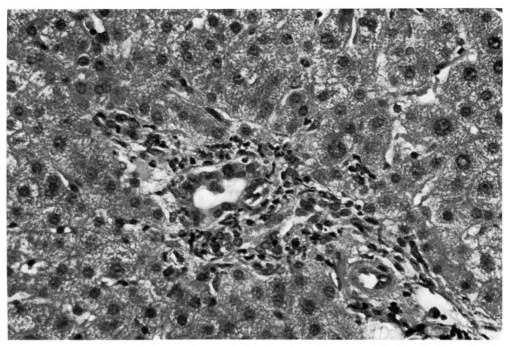

Fig. 20: Portal tract with slight, mainly marginal infiltration with neutrophils. The limiting plate is preserved and the liver cells appear normal (Needle biopsy, H & E x 270).

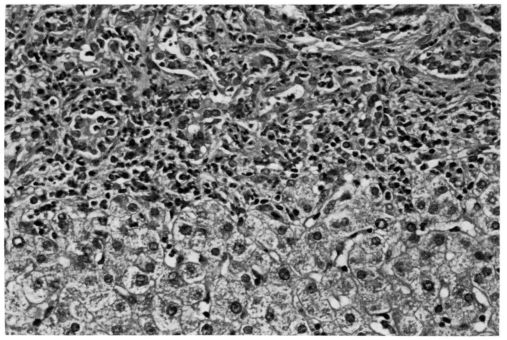

Fig. 21: Part of enlarged portal tract with marginal bile duct proliferation and a moderate-severe mainly marginal infiltration by neutrophils. There are multiple small defects of the limiting plate (Needle biopsy, H & E x 270).

Predominance of lymphocytes

Morphology: The most frequently encountered inflammatory cell in the portal tracts is the small lymphocyte. It may, when the inflammation is slight, be the only cell present. However, as pointed out previously, it is very exceptional to find only one type of inflammatory cell, and there are nearly always other cells such as histiocytes and plasma cells (Fig. 22) or possibly neutrophils.

Infiltration with predominance of lymphocytes can be of all grades of severity. The infiltration is usually most pronounced in the central parts of the portal tracts and diminishes towards the periphery[234, 236]. If the inflammation is very dense, it may be difficult to distinguish structures such as vessels and bile ducts.

If the inflammation is severe in the peripheral parts of the portal tracts also, there are often lymphocytes in the periportal parts of the lobules, so-called spillover[31](Fig. 23).

Morphological diagnosis: Under the light microscope lymphocytes are identified by their size and by their nuclei, different from those of histiocytes and plasma cells.

In dense inflammatory cell infiltrates examined in H & E-stained sections it is, however, difficult or impossible in practice to differentiate lymphocytes from plasma cells and small histiocytes. It is recommended that methyl green pyronin, PAS after diastase and iron stains should also be used, the first for plasma cells and the other two for histiocytes.

Differential diagnosis: In our experience a few lymphocytes in the portal tracts are without pathological signifiance.

Infiltration by lymphocytes and infiltrates with predominance of lymphocytes in slight or moderate degrees is usually easy to distinguish from other cellular infiltrates. In contrast, dense inflammation chiefly consisting of lymphocytes may sometimes look somewhat similar to the infiltrates of chronic lymphatic leukemia or lymphosarcoma. In chronic lymphatic leukemia and lymphosarcoma the cellular density is, however, usually more pronounced, and the infiltrates are larger and often extend from the portal tracts into the parenchyma[248]. Furthermore the demarcation of the malignant infiltrates is nearly always more sharp than that of inflammatory infiltrates.

Additional morphological findings: Inflammation of the portal tracts with predominance of lymphocytes is seen in a variety of diseases inside and outside the liver, and consequently a great variety of additional morphological changes may arise. Most commonly the lobular changes are those of acute viral hepatitis or non-specific, reactive hepatitis (p. 180).

Even when the lymphocytic inflammation in the portal tracts is severe, the portal structures are most often preserved and normal. Yet in somes cases of primary biliary cirrhosis[69] and viral hepatitis[290] one may find abnormal bile duct epithelium, and in long-lasting inflammations such as chronic aggressive hepatitis periportal fibrosis develops[89].

Occurrence and significance: Inflammation of the portal tracts with lymphocytic predominance is very common, and is recorded in a high percentage of biopsies. Usually the inflammation is slight or moderate. If it is located centrally in the portal tracts and the parenchymal changes are non-specific, (i.e. a few dispersed focal liver cell necroses with focal Kupffer cell proliferation and possibly slight steatosis) the patient often has an extrahepatic disease such as peptic ulcer, gastric cancer, cholecystitis or pancreatitis[397]. A similar picture may also be present in a late stage of acute viral hepatitis[29].

When the lymphocytic inflammation in the portal tracts is severe and diffuse, chronic hepatitis is suspected, but severe portal lymphocytic inflammation is also often found in primary biliary cirrhosis[69, 325] and in drug addicts[187, 272].

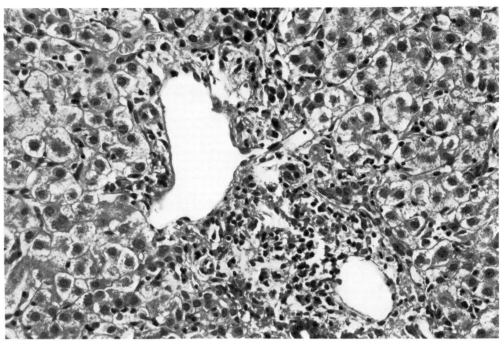

Fig. 22: Portal tract with a slight, diffuse infiltration with lymphocytes. There are in addition a few histiocytes and plasma cells (Needle biopsy, H & E x 270).

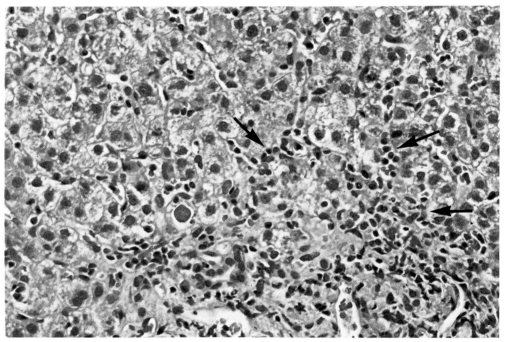

Fig. 23: Peripheral part of a portal tract with spillover indicated with arrows. A few acidophil bodies are seen close to and in the limiting plate (Needle biopsy, H & E x 270).

Predominance of plasma cells

Morphology: Infiltration of portal tracts by plasma cells is virtually always seen together with accumulation of lymphocytes and histiocytes[93] (Fig. 24). When the infiltration is slight it is usually diffusely distributed in the connective tissue, while the more severe forms are usually localized more in the periphery, with involvement of the periportal parenchyma[89, 251].

The plasma cells have a tendency to form small clusters (Fig. 25), and the most peripherally located ones are often seen in close relation to focal destruction of the limiting plate, as part of so-called piecemeal necrosis[89, 240] (p. 84).

Morphological diagnosis: When the inflammation is slight or moderate the identification of plasma cells is most often easy in H & E-stained sections, but in cases with severe inflammation and closely packed cells it may be impossible to differentiate plasma cells from lymphocytes and even histiocytes.

Staining for pyroninophilic substance is in such cases valuable, plasma cells being of characteristic size and form with typical, nuclear structure and location, and strongly pyroninophilic cytoplasm[41].

Differential diagnosis: Dense portal inflammation with predominance of plasma cells may be mistaken for inflammation with predominance of lymphocytes. Staining for pyroninophilic substance is usually very helpful[41].

In patients with myelomatosis, infiltrates of myeloma cells may be seen only in a minority of cases. These infiltrates are very closely packed and essentially without admixture of lymphocytes or histiocytes. The myeloma cells furthermore show cytologic signs of malignancy and there are nearly always other similar infiltrates in the parenchyma[115, 224].

Additional morphological findings: Many plasma cells in the peripheral parts of the portal tracts and in the periportal parts of the parenchyma are first and foremost seen in chronic aggressive hepatitis, especially in the more severe forms[89]. In these cases the central areas of the portal tracts are usually dominated by lymphocytes and histiocytes, and in some cases lymphoid follicles can be demonstrated. As a rule there are only few neutrophils. Except for the piecemeal necrosis the lobular changes are in most cases non-specific. However, lobular changes like those of acute viral hepatitis (p. 172) may be superimposed.

Many plasma cells in the peripheral parts of the portal tracts and periportally are also seen in some cases of acute viral hepatitis and are in such cases associated with the parenchymal changes of viral hepatitis[265].

Substantial numbers of plasma cells may in addition be found in primary biliary cirrhosis[69, 325], brucellosis[18], Wilson's disease[362] and other diseases.

A few plasma cells may be present in a great variety of conditions such as non-specific reactive hepatitis and large duct obstruction.

Occurrence and significance: The presence of a few plasma cells is thus very common and of no diagnostic significance.

Many plasma cells in the peripheral areas of the portal tracts together with substantial piecemeal necrosis lead in acute viral hepatitis to a suspicion of developing chronic aggressive hepatitis[101], and in chronic aggressive hepatitis their presence is an expression of histological activity with consequently greater chance of rapid development of cirrhosis[99].

The significance of large numbers of portal plasma cells in primary biliary cirrhosis[325] and Wilson's disease[362] is at present unknown.

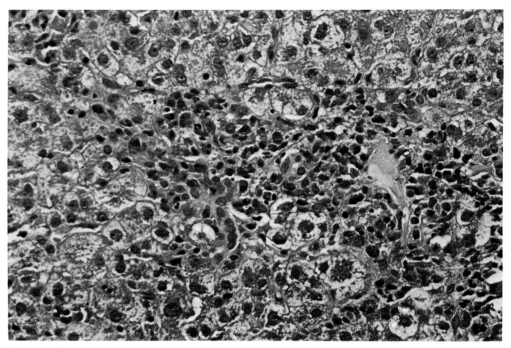

Fig. 24: Slightly enlarged portal tract with a mixed cellular infiltrate. There is a predominance of plasma cells (Needle biopsy, H & E x 270).

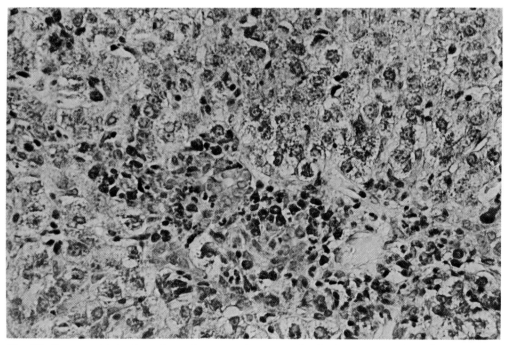

Fig. 25: Same portal tract as above demonstrating more clearly the great number of plasma cells. Note the tendency to cluster formation (Needle biopsy, Unna-Pappenheim x 270).

Predominance of eosinophils

Morphology: Eosinophils appear most often as scattered elements in portal inflammatory infiltrates (Fig. 26), but in some drug-induced liver lesions they can be the predominant or even the only inflammatory cells present[30, 187, 259, 272]. When predominant, the eosinophils are often situated in a varying number of smaller or larger groups without characteristic location in the portal tracts (Fig. 27).

When ramifications of the hepatic artery are encountered in polyarteriitis nodosa, many eosinophils together with neutrophils, lymphocytes, plasma cells, and histiocytes are to be found in and around the arterial walls[378, 400]. The inflammation may include part or all of the circumference.

Morphological diagnosis: Eosinophils are easily identified in H & E-stained sections. They are characterized by having two nuclear segments connected by a thick strand and by having large, strongly eosinophilic granules in the cytoplasm.

Differential diagnosis: On the assumption that H & E-staining is of adequate quality, infiltration with eosinophils offers no essential differential diagnostic problem.

Additional morphological findings: Scattered eosinophils in the portal tracts may be seen in a wide variety of diseases within and outside the liver, and many different parenchymal lesions can consequently be met. Examples are some cases of acute and chronic hepatitis and nonspecific reactive hepatitis. When a biopsy contains eosinophils in the portal tracts, one can often also demonstrate eosinophils in the parenchyma.

Predominance of eosinophils may be seen in a very few cases of acute hepatitis[265], but is more common in drug-induced lesion[30]. When a drug is the aetiologic factor, cholestasis in the parenchyma is frequently conspicuous[30].

In polyarteriitis nodosa one often finds other inflammatory cells as well as fibrinoid deposits and necrosis[400].

Occurrence and significance: The presence of a few eosinophils in the portal tracts is common and of no differential diagnostic significance. Portal eosinophils have been demonstrated in one third of our biopsies with acute viral hepatitis[265] and in one fifth with chronic aggressive hepatitis[58].

Predominance of eosinophils raises suspicion of a drug-induced liver disease[30, 187, 272], but may possibly be part of a virus-induced hepatitis[265].

Many eosinophils can furthermore be seen in parasitic infestations, e.g. schistosomiasis[5], and serial sections will probably disclose ova.

Eosinophils together with the other abovementioned changes in the arteries are diagnostic for polyarteriitis nodosa[400].

Finally it may be said that infiltrations of Hodgkins lymphoma as a rule comprise eosinophils[16].

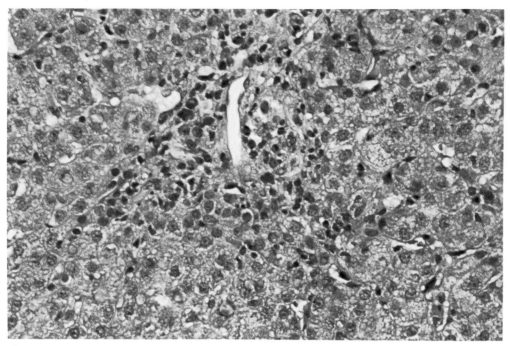

Fig. 26: Small portal tract with only slight infiltration of inflammatory cells. Scattered eosinophils are seen (Needle biopsy, H & E x 270).

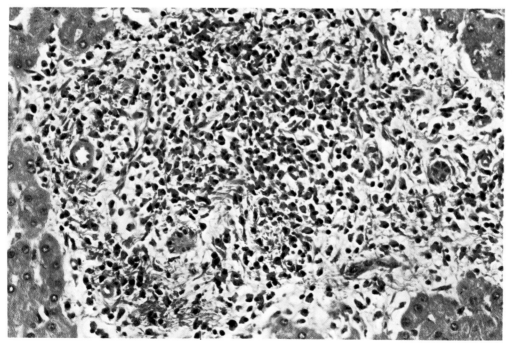

Fig. 27: Enlarged portal tract with a large inflammatory infiltrate with predominance of eosinophils (Surgical biopsy, H & E x 270).

Predominance of histiocytes

Morphology: Histiocytes are larger than lymphocytes and contain a weakly stained ovoid nucleus. After phagocytosis the cytoplasm acquires a characteristic appearance depending on the character of the material taken up. If the cells have phagocytosed ceroid, fine golden brown granules are seen in the cytoplasm[271]; the granules are deep red in PAS-stained sections after diastase digestion (Fig. 28). Haemosiderin granules are coarser and usually darker, and intensely blue in sections stained for iron[389] (Fig. 29).

More infrequently one may see malarial[110] or anthracotic pigments which are black, bile which is green (possibly greenblack or green-brown), thorotrast which is greyish-black and refractile[334], and copper which appears as tiny, dark granules in H & E-stained sections[205]. These are often very difficult to see without special staining procedures.

After phagocytosis of lipids the portal macrophages characteristically adapt the picture of lipophages. For discussion of epithelioid cells, see Granulomas, p. 42.

Histiocytes are usually seen diffusely distributed in the portal tracts, or they may have a tendency to form poorly demarcated groups which are without characteristic location. Histiocytes are nearly always found together with other inflammatory cells, especially lymphocytes and scanty neutrophils or plasma cells.

Morphological diagnosis: Histiocytes are in most cases relatively easy to recognize in H & E-stained sections, but for reliable differentiation from plasma cells, methyl green pyronin staining is recommended.

Moreover, staining for iron and with PAS after distase digestion is recommended routinely in order to differentiate between the two most commonly found types of histiocytes.

Differential diagnosis: As indicated above we prefer three special stains in the daily routine in order to distinguish histiocytes from plasma cells and to recognize histiocytes with phagocytized ceroid and iron, respectively. The differentiation of other types of histiocytes may require additional procedures.

Additional morphological findings: Histiocytes may, like lymphocytes, be found in a large number of diseases within and outside the liver, and the presence of these cells in the portal tracts may consequently be associated with many different morphological changes in the parenchyma.

Occurrence and significance: Slight inflammation dominated by histiocytes is common and nonspecific.

More pronounced inflammation with many histiocytes, often with PAS-positive diastase-resistant granules in the cytoplasm, is a constant phenomenon in the fully developed and especially late stage of acute viral hepatitis[265]. In approximately half of the cases with hepatitis iron-positive granules are also seen[265]. Demonstration of ceroid and iron-loaded histiocytes is important in the differentiation from non-specific hepatitis[289] (p. 180).

Histiocyte-dominated inflammation is moreover typical for chronic persistent hepatis[58, 89] (p. 178).

In infectious mononucleosis there is, in addition to lobular changes (p. 182), often a very dense portal infiltration with mononuclear elements, usually with some variation in the form and the stainability of the nuclei[17, 387].

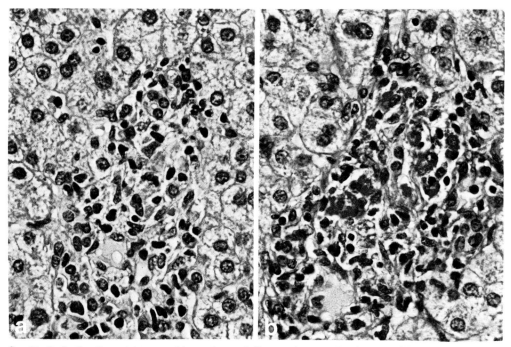

fig. 28: Left. Small portal tract with moderate inflammation, predominance of histiocytes (Needle biopsy, H & E x 400). Right. Same portal tract demonstrating ceroid pigment in histiocytes (PAS after diastase x 400).

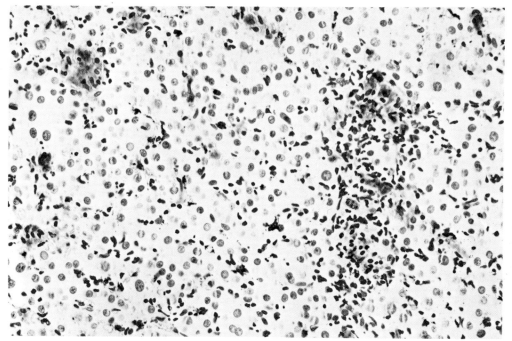

Fig. 29: Part of lobule from a patient with acute hepatitis. Iron-containing pigment in both parenchymal and portal histiocytes is conspicuous (Needle biopsy, Perls' stain x 110).

Granulomas and lymfoid follicles

Morphology: A granuloma is here defined as a compact, rounded collection of histiocytes not necessarily accompanied by other features such as necrosis[2]. Most granulomas in the portal tracts are epithelioid cell granulomas[190]. Such granulomas may be small, but are as a rule 100–200 µm in diameter. Usually the biopsy contains many granulomas, and they are to be found in all areas of the portal tracts and may also involve the lobule[131, 190].

Epithelioid cell granulomas and other granulomas in the liver do not differ essentially from granulomas elsewhere (Fig. 30). Epithelioid cell granulomas in miliary tuberculosis do, however, show conspicuous caseous necrosis only in relatively few cases, and it is often not possible to demonstrate acidfast bacilli[131]. Similarly, it is only occasionally possible to demonstrate doubly refractive crystals in narcotics. Specific structures, such as ova of Schistosoma mansoni, are present in the relevant specific diseases[5].

Most granulomas in the liver are infiltrated by lymphocytes, plasma cells and fibroblasts and are surrounded by collagen fibers with concentric structure in the early stages. When the granulomas are healed, a small, often hyalinized, fibrotic nodule may be demonstrated[216].

Lymphoid follicles with or without germinal centers are sometimes seen in portal tracts. In addition to lymphocytes, plasma cells and histiocytes are usually present. The follicles have a central position in the portal tracts, most often in close relation to a bile duct[59] (Fig. 31). In a needle biopsy they are usually scanty.

Morphological diagnosis: Both granulomas and lymphoid follicles are as a rule easily recognized in H & E-stained sections. In doubtful cases serial sections are in our experience very valuable. For instance, the presence of giant cells nearly always heralds granulomas deeper in the block. Sections stained for reticulin most often give an indication of the presence of granulomas and lymphoid follicles even at low magnification, since these lesions contain little or no reticulin.

Differential diagnosis: Granulomas are virtually never difficult to identify. Most portal granulomas are found in sarcoidosis[168], but it is always wise to examine Ziehl-Neelsen and PAS stains and to evaluate the lesion in polarized light. We have never seen lipogranulomas (p. 94) in the portal tracts[57].

Additional morphological findings: Epithelioid cell granulomas are as a rule associated with nonspecific chronic inflammatory changes[170], but may also be found in acute[265] and chronic hepatitis[58] and cirrhosis. In unusual cases of sarcoidosis with very numerous granulomas, cirrhosis may develop[216].

Granulomas with a very close relationship to the larger bile ducts are characteristic for early lesion of primary biliary cirrhosis[69, 325].

Lymphoid follicles are found particularly in chronic aggressive hepatitis[58, 59], and only rarely in acute hepatitis[290] or cirrhosis. Germinal centers are found mainly in the same portal tracts as, and in close relation to, bile ducts with abnormal epithelium[59].

Occurrence and significance: In large collections of liver biopsies, granulomas are found in less than 1 per cent[170, 190]. They are most frequently found in biopsies from patients with sarcoidosis[168], primary biliary cirrhosis[325], and miliary tuberculosis[150]. In drug addicts with acute hepatitis granulomas are found in approximately 5–10 per cent[265]. Granulomas may in addition be found in many other conditions. Examples are: brucellosis[18], beryllosis, schistosomiasis[5], syphilis[198], gastrointestinal malignant disease[190], drug lesion[187], ulcerative colitis and Crohn's disease[106]. The most common drugs are sulphonamides[127], phenylbutazone[146], halothane[105], steroids[187], and allopurinol[187]. The etiology can not always be elucidated.

Lymphoid follicles are uncommon, and they always indicate the need for a search for bile ducts with abnormal epithelium[59].

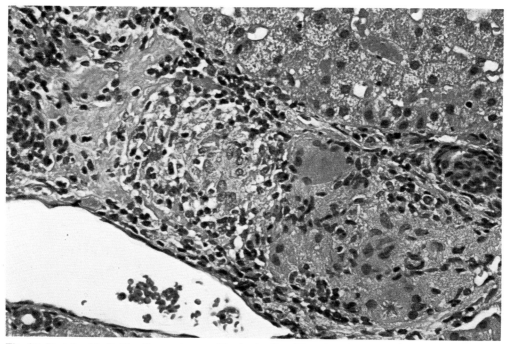

Fig. 30: Portal epithelioid cell granuloma with giant cells of Langhans' type. A characteristic asteroid body is seen at lower right and an area of hyaline fibrosis at upper left. The patient had sarcoidosis (Needle biopsy, H & E x 270).

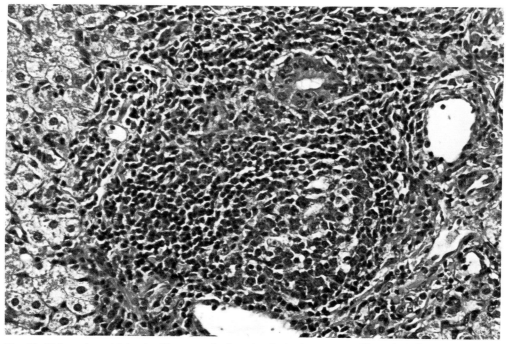

Fig. 31: Enlarged portal tract with a germinal center in its lower part. There is inflammation with many lymphocytes and plasma cells. Serial sections disclosed abnormal bile duct epithelium in the same duct as shown here (Needle biopsy, H & E x 270).

Edema

Morphology: Edema of the portal tracts is usually localized mainly to the peripheral areas of the connective tissue[67, 291]. The tissue has a looser structure than normal with increased distance between the bundles of collagen and splitting up of the individual bundles. In addition there is in H & E-stained sections a diffuse bluish-slate tint (Fig. 32 & 33). In the same areas infiltration with neutrophils and so-called marginal bile duct proliferation are commonly found. As a rule most or all portal tracts are involved, but the edema may vary widely in degree[291].

Less often the edema is predominantly in the central parts of the portal tracts, around bile ducts. In such cases the bile duct epithelium is often abnormal, and it is important to follow these changes in serial sections[69].

Morphological diagnosis: Edema is best recognized in H & E-stained sections, and the simultaneous occurrence of a bluish tint and splitting up of the collagen bundles usually leads to correct identification. Mild degrees of edema may, however, be difficult to establish, especially in poorly processed slides.

Differential diagnosis: Slight edema may easily be overlooked, but in most cases the diagnosis is easy and without differential diagnostic problems.

Additional morphological findings: Edema of the peripheral parts of the portal tracts is first and foremost met with in patients with obstruction of the larger bile ducts[67, 291]. Besides portal changes with edema, infiltration of neutrophils and marginal bile duct proliferation, centrilobular cholestasis is found in the parenchyma. In the early stages the cholestasis is "pure", but later liver cells may undergo focal necrosis.

Edema, often associated with similar portal changes, may also be seen in some cases of alcoholic hepatitis[66] and acute hepatitis caused by virus or drugs, especially when there is pronounced cholestasis[29]. Alcoholic hepatitis is characterized by Mallory bodies, liver cell necrosis and neutrophils[56], while acidophil bodies, focal liver cell necrosis, focal Kupffer cell proliferation and ballooning are constant features in acute hepatitis of viral type[29].

Edema around the centrally situated portal bile ducts may be found in primary biliary cirrhosis[69] and in large duct obstruction[291].

Occurrence and significance: Edema of the connective tissue of the portal tracts has been recorded in 5–10 per cent of the biopsies in our material, but the exact frequency clearly depends on the nature of the series.

Edema of portal tracts is always accociated with other changes. In most cases the diagnosis is large bile duct obstruction[67, 291], but a careful evalution of both portal tracts and parenchyma is necessary in order to exclude other diagnosis such as hepatitis[29].

Edema of the portal tracts is thus not a pathognomonic lesion.

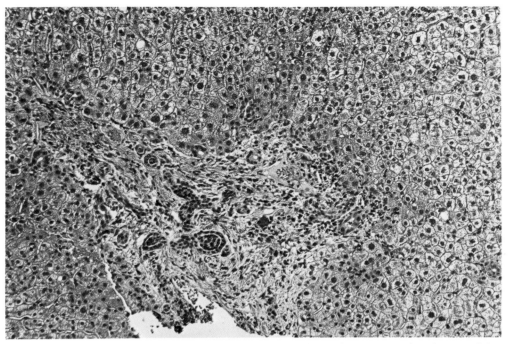

Fig. 32: Survey of an enlarged portal tract with a slate-colored, loose connective tissue mainly in its lower and right part. The slate color represents the edema (from a patient with large duct obstruction) (Needle biopsy, H & E x 110).

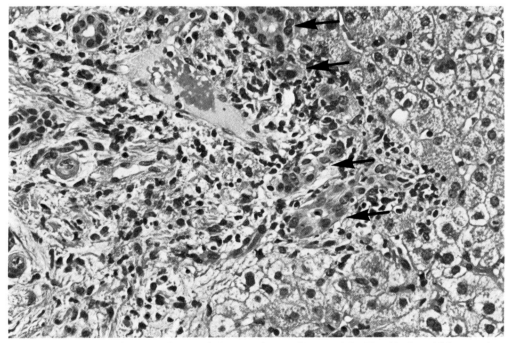

Fig. 33: Higher magnification of part of the portal tract illustrated in Fig. 32. In addition to the edema, inflammation with many neutrophils and marginal bile duct proliferation are visible (arrows) (Needle biopsy, H & E x 270).

Decreased number

Morphology: The smallest portal tracts normally contain one bile duct, and the medium sized portal tracts two or three[156, 160]. A decreased number of interlobular and septal bile ducts may be found in so-called intrahepatic biliary atresia[171] and in the later stages of primary biliary cirrhosis[279, 325].

The term intrahepatic biliary atresia[171] does not fit correctly with the now generally accepted theory that the primary lesion is destructive rather than developmental. In the early stages necrosis of the bile duct epithelium has been described, whereas the later stages are characterized by a reduced number of centrally located bile ducts in the portal tracts, and fibrosis with lipophages.

In the early stages of primary biliary cirrhosis the most prominent changes are necrosis and degeneration of the epithelium, mainly of septal bile ducts. Inflammation and often granulomatous reactions are also present[69] (p. 56). Later the central areas of the affected portal tracts show fibrosis (Fig. 34), sometimes with atrophic remnants or the original bile ducts[325] (Fig. 35).

Morphological diagnosis: It may be difficult even in serial sections to prove that the number of portal bile ducts is decreased. If a needle biopsy from a normal liver contains only tangentially cut portal tracts, the number of recognizable bile ducts is small, even in large specimens.

In intrahepatic biliary atresia it is difficult or impossible to identify the remnants of the original duct system. The morphological relations are further complicated by the fact that it is sometimes difficult to demonstrate portal bile ducts even in normal neonatal liver tissue[171].

If a biopsy comprises parts of the intrahepatic biliary tree showing retrograde changes and inflammation, it is diagnostic for destructive intrahepatic bile duct disease[340, 373]. If the changes have progressed to atrophy and fibrosis, they are more difficult to diagnose. Serial sections with demonstration of fibrosis corresponding to the original biliary tree, possibly with inflammation or with transition to preserved segments of the tree, sometimes enable a diagnosis of primary biliary cirrhosis to be made[279, 325].

Differential diagnosis: As indicated above, it is often not easy to prove a decrease in the number of portal bile ducts, even with the use of serial sections. The greatest diagnostic security is achieved when retrograde changes of the epithelium also are present.

Additional morphological findings: In early stages of intrahepatic biliary atresia there are, in addition to the portal changes cholestasis, focal liver cell necrosis, and inflammation. Giant liver cells may be found in the lobules. Later biliary cirrhosis develops[171].

In the early stages of primary biliary cirrhosis the lobular changes are usually slight and non-characteristic, with focal liver cell necrosis and Kupffer cell proliferation. Cholestasis it most often absent[69, 325]. Piecemeal necrosis may be present. Later the smallest portal tracts may show signs of obstruction of the larger branches of the biliary tree with marginal bile duct proliferation, edema, and neutrophils[69, 325] (Fig. 34). Cirrhosis does not develop until late in the course of the disease[325] (p. 188).

Occurrence and significance: Both intrahepatic biliary atresia[171] and primary biliary cirrhosis[279] are uncommon diseases, and a diminished number of portal bile ducts is consequently not a frequent phenomenon in most series. The morphological diagnosis of decreased numbers of portal bile ducts is not easily made, unless retrograde epithelial changes are also demonstrable. A suspicion of a decreased number of portal bile ducts renders primary biliary cirrhosis a possibility[325] and is an indication for the use of serial sections in order to demonstrate diagnostic features.

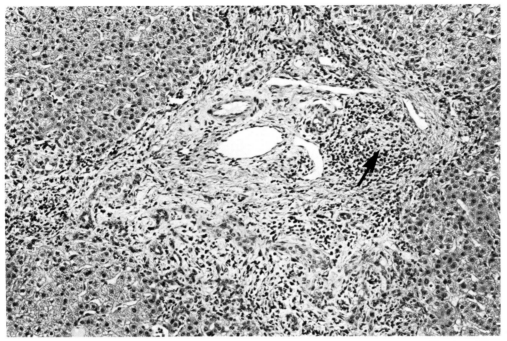

Fig. 34: Enlarged portal tract with edema, inflammation and marginal bile duct proliferation. The original bile duct is missing and replaced by a small scar (arrow) surrounded by lymphocytes (primary biliary cirrhosis) (Surgical biopsy, H & E x 110).

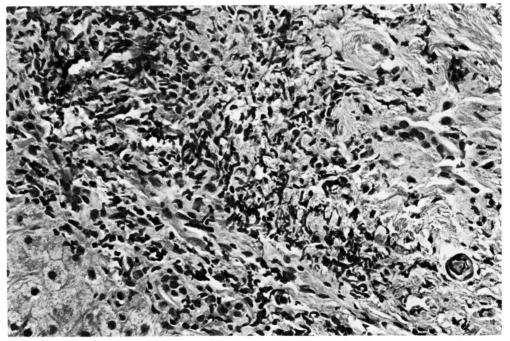

Fig. 35: High magnification of a similar lesion from another case of primary biliary cirrhosis. The scarified area with remnants of a bile duct is seen in the right half of the picture (Needle biopsy, H & E x 270).

Increased number – diffuse

Morphology: There are three causes of an increase in the visible number of bile ducts in the portal tracts. The first is an actual proliferation with new formation of bile ducts. The second is elongation and tortuousity of the original bile ducts, making them more conspicuous and transected more often (p. 50), and the third is a congenital anomaly with more bile ducts than normal (p. 52).

True bile duct proliferation can be found in all degrees of severity (Fig. 36 & 37). When the lobular architecture is preserved, the proliferation is usually only slight or moderate[29, 89, 291], whereas it is often pronounced in cirrhosis[225]. When the proliferation is mild it may be localized to a few portal tracts, but most often it is seen to varying degrees in most portal tracts.

The smallest proliferating ducts have cuboidal epithelium, the larger cuboidal or columnar epithelium[225, 359]. Both the nuclei and the cytoplasm are darker than in the corresponding normal epithelium.

Bile duct proliferation may be diffusely distributed throughout the portal tracts[359] or mainly localized to the peripheral areas (so-called marginal bile duct proliferation)[291]. On this page the diffuse type is discussed.

Morphological diagnosis: The diagnosis is usually easy. When proliferation is minimal, it may be difficult to distinguish from normal. Evaluation of many portal tracts and use of serial sections are necessary.

When portal inflammation is severe, the diagnosis may also be difficult, in that it may not be easy to distinguish small proliferating ducts from groups of closely set histiocytes. Reticulin staining with demonstration of the concentric reticulin network, or PAS staining with demonstration of basement membrane material is usually helpful.

Differential diagnosis: As indicated above, the identification of diffuse bile duct proliferation is as a rule easy. When the number of bile ducts is increased because of a congenital anomaly, the ducts are larger and have a more irregular outline, and they are set in more abundant and more mature connective tissue (p. 52).

Additional morphological findings: Diffuse bile duct proliferation is found in many different liver diseases, and the lesion may therefore be associated with various parenchymal and portal changes. Significant bile duct proliferation is characteristic of chronic aggressive hepatitis[89] and cirrhosis[225]. Slight proliferation is to be demonstrated in a substantial number of cases of acute hepatitis later in the disease[265].

In other diseases with pronounced inflammation in the portal connective tissue, diffuse bile duct proliferations may also be seen. Examples are ascending cholangitis[340, 373] and mucoviscidosis[381].

Occurrence and significance: Diffuse bile duct proliferation is a frequent and non-specific change which is found mainly in association with pronounced portal inflammation. Increased amounts of connective tissue in the liver especially periportal fibrosis are similarly often seen together with bile duct proliferation.

The slight diffuse portal bile duct proliferation typically seen in acute viral hepatitis is reversible[331].

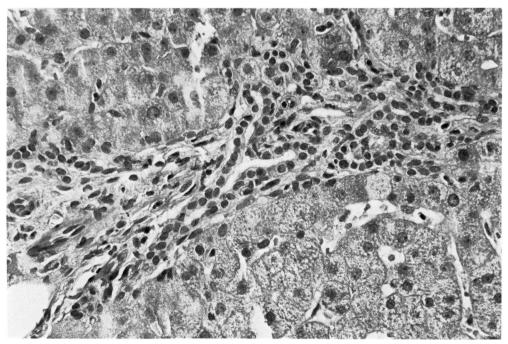

Fig. 36: Part of slightly enlarged medium-sized portal tract with slight fibrosis and slight, diffuse increase in the number of bile ducts. The limiting plate is preserved (Needle biopsy, H & E x 270).

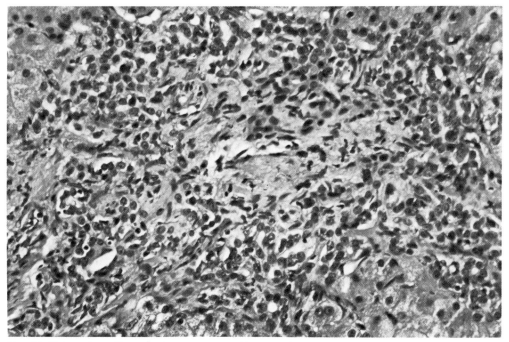

Fig. 37: Enlarged medium-sized portal tract with some fibrosis and a pronounced increase in the number of bile ducts. The bile ducts are diffusely distributed (Needle biopsy, H & E x 270).

Increased number – marginal

Morphology: So-called marginal bile duct proliferation consists in the early stages of hyperplasia of the epithelium of ducts located at the periphery of the portal tracts. The lumen of the ducts is rounded or serpiginous, and delineated by a cuboidal or columnar epithelium[67, 291]. In many cases longitudinally cut ducts are prominent; these have an intimate relation to the liver cells in the limiting plate (Fig. 38). Edema of the adjacent connective tissue and infiltration with neutrophils are very common[291].

This elongation of the original ducts may be followed by actual duct proliferation with destruction of the limiting plates and sometimes fibrosis. Marginal bile duct proliferation is usually present in most or all portal tracts in a biopsy[291], but may, depending on the primary disease, be confined to one or a few tracts. The lesion is usually confined to only a part of the affected tract (Fig. 39).

It is common to find disperse retrograde changes in the epithelial cells of the proliferating ducts with karyopyknosis and swelling of the cytoplasm. Neutrophils may be seen in the ducts in relation to areas of necrosis[291].

Morphological diagnosis: When the number of marginally located bile ducts is markedly increased, the diagnosis is easy even in H & E-stained sections. When the increase is only slight, it is very important to use serial sections, some of which should be stained for reticulin and collagen fibers.

Differential diagnosis: Marginal bile duct proliferation is distinguished from diffuse bile duct proliferation mainly by its location. Both forms, however, may be seen simultaneously. Marginal bile duct proliferation is often followed by retrograde epithelial changes, edema, and infiltration with neutrophils[291].

Additional morphological findings: Marginal bile duct proliferation is seen mainly in biopsies from patients with obstruction of the biliary tree[291] or acute hepatitis (virus – or drug – induced) with pronounced cholestasis[29].

In the early stages of large duct obstruction the lobular changes are minimal except for cholestasis. In longstanding obstruction focal liver cell necrosis and inflammation arise in relation to the bile thrombi[291].

In most examples of hepatitis the parenchymal changes are typical. In a few cases the lobular changes, i.e. necrosis, ballooning and inflammation, may be slight and these cases are more difficult to distinguish from large bile duct obstruction (p. 186).

It is also important to know that marginal bile duct proliferation is sometimes found in biopsies from alcoholics[66]. A picture of alcoholic hepatitis is usually seen in the parenchyma.

Occurrence and significance: Marginal bile duct proliferation is recorded in 5–10 per cent of our biopsies. The finding is so constant in large duct obstruction that if absent in a well-processed biopsy with more than 10 to 12 portal tracts, this diagnosis can be excluded[291].

Marginal bile duct proliferation is furthermore often seen in smaller portal tracts in biopsies from patients with obstructive disease in the larger intrahepatic ducts, such as primary biliary cirrhosis[69], biliary atresia and mucoviscidosis. The same change may be found locally when tumors, commonly metastases, compress ducts.

When marginal bile duct proliferation is conspicuous in acute hepatitis, cholestasis is often prominent, and when this type of proliferation is seen in alcoholics, pancreatitis is usually demonstrable[333].

Marginal bile duct proliferation, together with other portal and parenchymal changes, is a very important factor in determining the etiology of cholestasis[291].

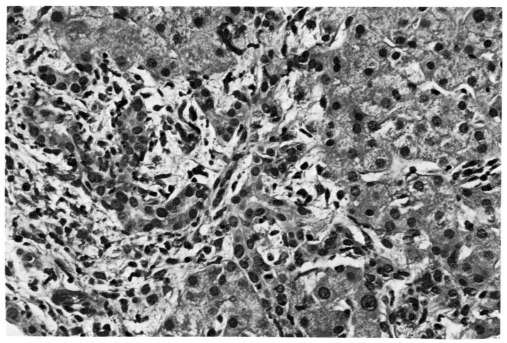

Fig. 38: Peripheral part of a large portal tract showing pronounced edema, moderate inflammation and characteristic bile duct proliferation (marginal). The epithelium of the ducts is cuboidal or low columnar (Needle biopsy, H & E x 270).

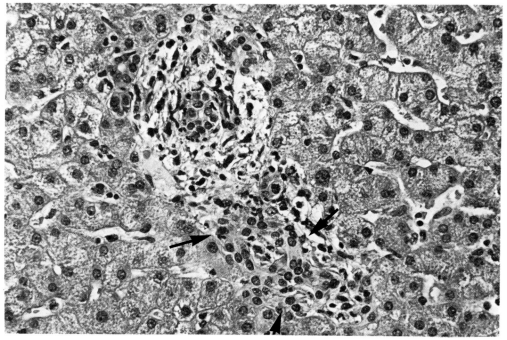

Fig. 39: Small portal tract with edema and in its lower part with an area with prominent marginal bile duct proliferation (arrows). The inflammation is slight (Needle biopsy, H & E x 270).

Abnormal configuration

Morphology: Intrahepatic biliary atresia was previously thought to be congenital, but it is now widely accepted that the changes are secondary to an inflammatory reaction (p. 46). Two congenital bile duct anomalies will be described, the socalled ductal plate malformation[173] and cysts[232].

The ductal plate malformation consists three-dimensionally of a polygonal, plate-like lumen which is often curved, giving it a shield-like appearance. On both sides the lumen is covered by a single-layered, regular epithelium of bile duct type, columnar or cuboidal. This formation is always surrounded by abundant mature connective tissue[173]. Especially in serial sections one may find gradual transitions from the flat lumen to tubules. Similarly, obliterations of the flat lumen may be demonstrated, sometimes combined with cystic dilatation. The ductal plate malformation appears in a localized and a generalized form.

The localized form is called a *von Meyenburg's complex* or *microhamartoma* and appears in two-dimensional sections as a rounded lesion with many, usually slightly cystic lumina set in a uniformly mature connective tissue[232, 371] (Fig. 40). The complex is found in close relation to portal tracts, often between two or three tracts corresponding to branching points. There is as a rule no inflammation, but bile or eosinophilic material is often found in the lumina. The presence of two or three complexes in the same biopsy is not uncommon[371].

The generalized form is called *congenital hepatic fibrosis*[163, 183]. Enlarged fibrotic portal tracts are linked by fibrosis, which encircles the lobules (Fig. 41). In the connective tissue there are many slit-like, sometimes dilated bile ducts often containing inspissated bile thrombi.

Cysts may also appear in a localized and a generalized form. They are set in mature connective tissue and the epithelium is flat or cuboidal[232].

Morphological diagnosis: The identification of both the ductal plate malformation and the cysts is easy at low magnifications in H & E-stained sections.

Differential diagnosis: It is usually not difficult to distinguish the lesions in question from bile duct proliferation. The shape of the lumina and the presence of uniform mature connective tissue are of importance.

Additional morphological findings: Microhamartomas are usually incidental findings, and they can consequently be found together with all types of lesions[371]. The microhamartomas probably do not provoke secondary changes.

The lobular architecture is characteristically preserved in congenital hepatic fibrosis, but secondary changes such as infection (cholangitis)[163] and, rarely, cirrhosis may develop.

The above comments on the localized and generalized forms of the ductal plate malformation also apply to cysts.

Occurrence and significance: Microhamartomas have been demonstrated in less than 1 per cent of our biopsies[371]. When present in a biopsy it is probably always an expression of multiple lesions in the liver. They have scarcely any clinical significance and the same holds true for the non-generalized cysts.

Congenital hepatic fibrosis is uncommon. The most important clinical symptoms and signs are hepatomegaly and the sequelae of portal hypertension, e.g. hemorrhage from esophageal varices. The disease is as a rule diagnosed in the first and second decade of life, but sometimes it presents much later (50–60 years of age). Both congenital hepatic fibrosis and generalized cysts may be found together with cystic disease of kidneys and pancreas[183]. Congenital hepatic fibrosis is also described in Caroli's disease[163].

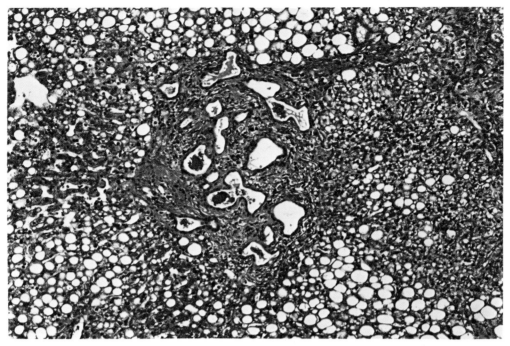

Fig. 40: Microhamartoma. In the center is a partly rounded area of mature connective tissue with numerous irregular bile duct structures, often with dilation and content of bile. The parenchyma is steatotic (Needle biopsy, H & E x 110).

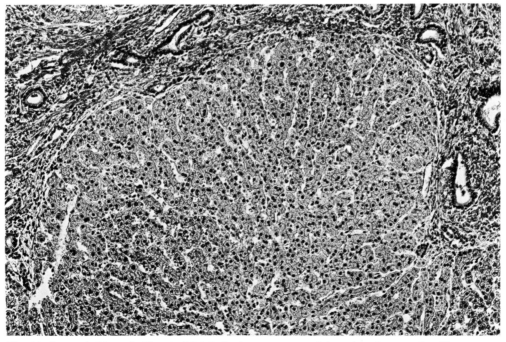

Fig. 41: Congenital hepatic fibrosis. Mainly in the upper part of the microphotograph a fibrous zone with many irregular bile ducts is demonstrated. The parenchyma shows preserved lobular architecture (Surgical biopsy, van Gieson x 110).

Abnormal epithelium – "hepatitis type"

Morphology: The epithelial cells of the affected portal bile ducts are swollen, more rounded than normal, sometimes being slightly polygonal. Their cytoplasm most often appears vacuolated (Fig. 42) but exceptionally it has an eosinophilic granular appearance. The nuclei may be hyperchromatic and the cellular limits blurred. The epithelium is nearly always multilayered, frequently having four to six prominent layers (Fig. 43). The lumen is often narrowed, but not occluded, and the outer diameter of the duct is increased. The epithelium and basement membrane are often lightly infiltrated by lymphocytes and plasma cells[69, 292].

The changes primarily involve medium-sized interlobular bile ducts situated in the centers of the portal tracts. The changes are segmental, often involving only part of the circumference of a duct. Usually only one or very few ducts with abnormal epithelium can be demonstrated in a needle biopsy specimen[292].

The connective tissue around the abnormal ducts is as a rule, but not always, severely or moderately infiltrated by lymphocytes, plasma cells, and histiocytes. Lymphoid follicles are sometimes found near the affected ducts, but granulomas have never been observed[292]. Periductal fibrosis is minimal or absent.

Morphological diagnosis: The diagnosis of this type of bile duct lesion is made only with certainty at high magnification. Under low power, the change is easily mistaken for inflammatory infiltration, particularly germinal centers in lymphoid follicles, or overlooked. Both H & E- and van Gieson-stained sections are helpful. Serial sections are of considerable value when in doubt, also to demonstrate the multifocal and segmental nature of the lesion.

Differential diagnosis: Abnormalities of the bile duct epithelium in portal tracts have been described in primary biliary cirrhosis (PBC)[69], drug reactions[401], large duct biliary obstruction[138, 291], and ulcerative colitis[283] and Crohn's disease[283], as well as in hepatitis[290] and posthepatic cirrhosis[294].

The typical PBC lesion of portal bile ducts is more uncommonly found in needle biopsies, since it is nearly always larger interlobular or segmental bile ducts which are affected[325]. In primary biliary cirrhosis the early changes in the portal bile ducts may resemble those described here, but in the majority of cases they are of a more destructive nature with rupture of the walls and with a granulomatous reaction in the adjacent connective tissue[69] (p. 56).

Changes in portal bile ducts have been described in a few cases of drug-induced hepatitis[401]. These are usually, but not always, marked by destruction and tend to affect the smaller portal ducts.

The karyopyknosis and variation in size and polarity of bile duct epithelium in large-duct biliary obstruction is seen in the proliferating small ducts at the margins of the portal tracts[67].

In rare cases of ulcerative colitis and Crohn's disease a lesion of the portal ducts resembling the early lesion of PBC has been described[283].

Additional morphological findings: This bile duct lesion has been demonstrated in acute viral hepatitis[290], chronic persistent hepatitis[58], chronic aggressive hepatitis[59] and cirrhosis[294].

Occurrence and significance: Whereas we have found only very few cases of acute viral hepatitis[290] and chronic persistent hepatitis cases[58] with abnormal bile duct epithelium, the lesion is encountered in approximately 35–40 per cent of all cases of chronic aggressive hepatitis[59] and approximately 7 per cent of all cirrhosis cases[294]. Patients with acute viral hepatitis with abnormal bile duct epithelium more often develop chronic hepatitis than patients without abnormal bile ducts[71], and patients with chronic aggressive hepatitis with abnormal ducts develop cirrhosis more quickly and more frequently than similar patients without abnormal ducts[59].

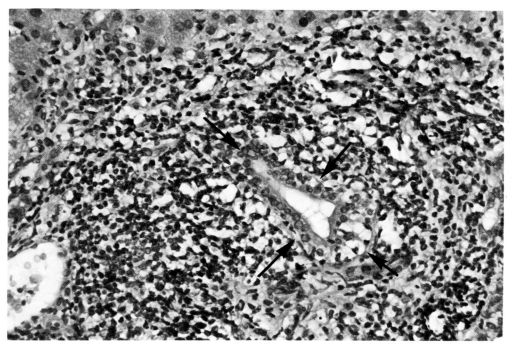

Fig. 42: Part of medium-sized portal tract with moderate inflammation and a bile duct with vacuolated partly multilayered epithelium. The basement membrane of the duct is indicated by arrows. From a case of chronic aggressive hepatitis (Needle biopsy, H & E x 270).

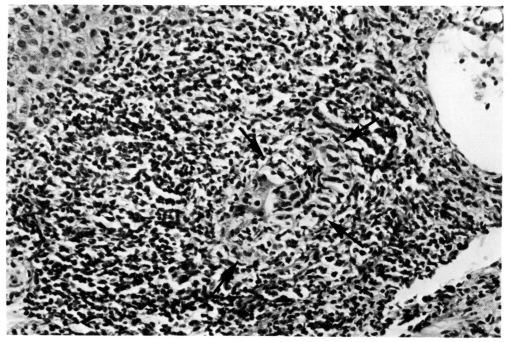

Fig. 43: Part of medium-sized portal tract with severe inflammation and a severely damaged bile duct with vacoulation and stratification (arrows). Left of the abnormal duct a lymphoid follicle is seen. From another case of CAH (Needle biopsy, van Gieson x 270).

Abnormal epithelium – "PBC-type"

Morphology: In primary biliary cirrhosis (PBC, p. 188) the affected parts of the biliary tree are primarily the septal and larger interlobular ducts with a central position in the portal tracts. The cells are swollen with a finely granular, eosinophillic cytoplasm and little or no vacuolation. They are arranged in a single layer, but are often crowded or compressed and have blurred borders (Fig. 44). The nuclei may be pyknotic. The basement membrane is in places indistinct, and complete rupture may also occur (Fig. 45). The lumen contains cells, debris, or mucin. The epithelium is only rarely infiltrated by inflammatory cells, but the lesion is surrounded by a loose infiltrate of lymphocytes, histiocytes and plasma cells. Also a few eosinophils may be present. Germinal centers are rare, but epithelioid cell granulomas are frequent. The granulomas, which sometimes contain giant cells, are located close to the ducts with abnormal epithelium and sometimes envelop them (Fig. 44). Serial sections show that the duct lesions are segmental and usually involve the whole circumference[69, 93, 153, 279, 325].

The portal tracts with abnormal ducts often contain in addition proliferating smaller bile ducts with marginal localization, accompanied by neutrophils[69]. Later, the portal tracts show both diffuse and periductal fibrosis, the latter sometimes annular in type. In some cases the fibrosis surrounds a partly or totally atrophic duct[279, 325].

Morphological diagnosis: The typical early lesion is easily recognized in H & E-stained sections, whereas staining for collagen fibers is to be recommended in the later stages. It is important that serial sections should be examined in all cases suspected of this type of lesion.

As indicated above the changes primarily involve septal and large interlobular ducts. The diagnosis can therefore often be made only in surgical biopsies, since such relatively large ducts may be absent from needly biopsy specimens.

Differential diagnosis: This type of bile duct lesion is in most cases typical but there are several points of similarity to the bile duct lesion of hepatitis[69]. The latter is characterized by vacuolation and proliferation of the epithelium, but both granular epithelium and destructions are sometimes found. The PBC lesion affects larger ducts and is often accompanied by granulomas, and lymphoid follicles are less often seen[69].

Additional morphological findings: In the larger portal tracts there is virtually always some degree of inflammation dominated by scattered lymphocytes and histiocytes. Epithelioid cell granulomas are common. Furthermore piecemeal necrosis may be present. In the early stages there is only minimal parenchymal damage and usually no cholestasis[69].

Marginal bile duct proliferation, edema and neutrophils are often demonstrated in smaller portal tracts, without changes in bile duct epithelium. This change is probably caused by obstruction of the larger branches of the biliary tree by the lesion in question[69].

In the later stages of PBC the amount of connective tissue increases and parenchymal nodules may develop. The cirrhosis is characterized by a decreased number of original bile ducts (but an increase in newly formed smaller ducts) and parenchymal cholestasis[279, 325].

Occurrence and significance: No exact figures are available as to the frequency of this lesion, but it is usually refered to as rare. There is, however, no doubt that the lesion is underdiagnosed. We find the bile duct change in 1–2 per cent of our biopsies with the help of routine serial sections.

The great majority of patients with this change have primary biliary cirrhosis, but a similar lesion, may be seen in some patients with ulcerative colitis or Crohn's disease[283], and in some cases of drug reaction (for instance due to barbiturates and chlorpromazine)[401].

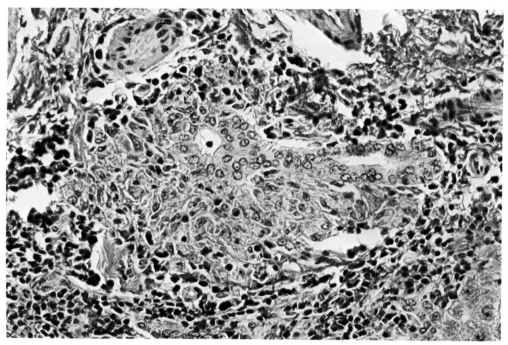

Fig. 44: Part of large portal tract with a longitudinally cut bile duct (center). The epithelial cells are slightly enlarged and in the left side the cellular outlines are blurred, and an early epithelioid cell granuloma is present (PBC) (Surgical biopsy, van Gieson x 270).

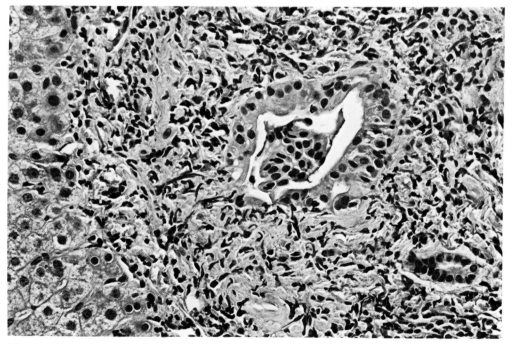

Fig. 45: Part of large portal tract with an abnormal bile duct (PBC). In the lower left part of the duct the cells are atrophic or missing. Around the duct, fibrosis with inflammation and scattered epitheliod cells is found (Surgical biopsy, H & E x 270).

Pigments

Morphology: The most commonly found pigments in the portal tracts are ceroid and iron. Less common is bile, and other pigments such as carbon, thorotrast and malarial pigment are only rarely seen.

Ceroid is a golden brown pigment, which in portal tracts is present in histiocytes as fine granules (Fig. 28). It is first seen in sinusoidal histiocytes. These move from the parenchyma to the portal tracts, and are arranged in groups or singly[28, 96]. *Iron* is seen as fine, dark brown granules most often in histiocytes, but sometimes also extracellularly in the connective tissue, in vessel walls or in bile duct epithelium. It is often found together with ceroid in histiocytes[265]. *Bile* pigment in portal tracts may be in the form of bile thrombi in ducts or as small clumps within histiocytes[327c]. Bile pigment varies in color and texture, but usually bile in histiocytes is green, sometimes with a brownish tinge, whereas bile plugs in ducts are larger and usually dark green to black. In very rare cases a bile lake is formed from leakage of large amounts of bile from a duct. Around the extravasate there is inflammation, often with foreign body giant cells[327e] (Fig. 46). *Carbon* is seen as minute black granules, *thorotrast* as birefringent, greyish, irregular granules[334] (Fig. 47) and *malarial*[110] and *schistosomial pigment*[5] as dark brown to black granules.

Morphological diagnosis: Although ceroid and iron can be recognized in H & E-stained sections, it is easier and safer to identify and differentiate them with special stain, e.g. PAS after diastase for ceroid and Perls' stain for iron. The latter method, and the van Gieson stain are excellent even for the recognition of minute amounts of bile pigment.

Differential diagnosis: Differentiation between ceroid and iron containing pigment calls for special stains (see above).

Bile granules may be difficult to differentiate from ceroid but bile is most often negative or only weakly stained with PAS after diastase and in Perls' and van Gieson's stains the green color is conspicuous.

Carbon is completely black. It may be very similar to silver granules but the latter is situated mainly extracellularly. Thorotrast is easily diagnosed when one is familiar with the picture. The malarial pigment is more brownish than carbon.

Additional morphological findings: Clumps of ceroid – containing histiocytes are usually seen in acute or chronis aggressive hepatitis[29, 97], but smaller numbers of such cells are very common.

Clumps of histiocytes with iron-positive granules are most often associated with acute hepatitis[29]. Iron in the connective tissue, vessels and bile ducts mainly occurs in connection with fibrosis or cirrhosis[180].

Occurrence and significance: Small amounts of ceroid in portal histiocytes are a very common finding and without diagnostic significance. In contrast, clumps of ceroid-containing histiocytes are a constant phenomenon in acute hepatitis (viral or drug-induced) in the fully developed and late stages[29]. Clumps of histiocytes with iron-positive pigment are found in approximately half of cases of acute hepatitis, mainly in the late stage[265].

Iron in the connective tissue, vessels and bile ducts is most typically seen in hemochromatosis[180] but the amount of iron may also be very high, for instance, in some alcoholics[54, 393].

The presence of carbon is very rare. It is an expression of anastomosis between thoracic and abdominal lymph and speaks in favor of an altered mediastinal lymph flow.

Thorotrast is also rare. In our material it is found in a few patients in whom X-ray examinations were performed with the now obsolete thorotrast as contrast medium[384].

Malarial and schistosomial pigment in portal histiocytes is usually found together with hyperplasia of and pigment in Kupffer cells[5, 110]. The two pigments closely resemble each other and the differentiation is to be made on other criteria.

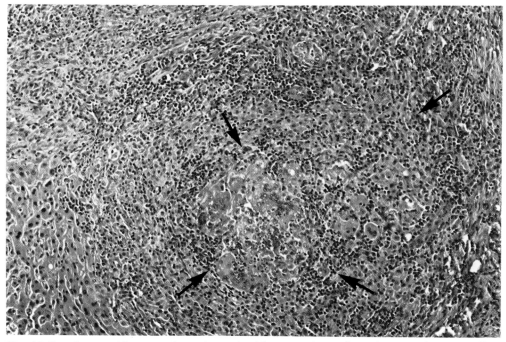

Fig. 46: Portal tract with a granuloma (arrows) with many giant cells and a central orange-yellow precipitate (bile lake). There is a conspicuous inflammatory infiltrate with resulting compression of the adjacent parenchyma (lower left) (Surgical biopsy, H & E x 270).

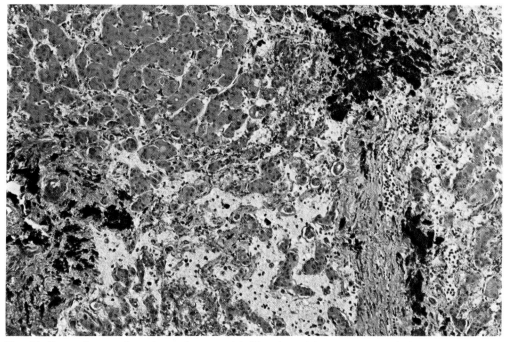

Fig. 47: Parts of two enlarged portal tracts with fibrosis and large amounts of thorotrast pigment. The pigment is seen as irregular granules or clumps of granules. In the parenchyma irregular sinusoidal dilatation is found (Surgical biopsy, H & E x 110).

Vessels

Morphology: Changes in portal vessels are relatively uncommon, but may be found in branches of both the hepatic artery and the portal vein. *Arteries:* The most frequent lesion is arteriolosclerosis with homogeneous thickening of the subendothelial layer. The lumen is narrowed but without thrombosis, and there is no inflammatory reaction[20, 327i] (Fig. 48).

In polyarteriitis nodosa the alterations mainly affect the arteries in the larger portal tracts. In typical cases fibrinoid with necrosis as well as inflammatory cells are seen throughout the wall. Neutrophils and eosinophils are often the predominant cells. Thrombosis is frequent. As elsewhere the lesion is segmental, and serial sections are important. In non-typical cases only foci of inflammation may be seen[51, 400].

Amyloid deposits are also similar to those in other tissues. The material is present as a homogenous eosinophilic layer in the subendothelial zone, and when sparse, it may be overlooked in routine stain[357].

Thrombotic material is usually seen together with inflammation of the wall (polyarteriitis nodosa) but may also arise in otherwise normal arteries[51]. *Veins:* Thrombosis of the portal vein branches (Fig. 49) may complicate cirrhosis, particularly when hepatocellular carcinoma invades the veins[111a]. In acute pylephlebitis septic thrombi are seen, often accompanied by neutrophils in the vessel wall[339].

Granulomas in vein walls are seen in schistosomiasis with ova, and in larger branches adult worms may be demonstrated[5].

In very rare instances smaller portal vein branches show thickening and an inconspicuous lumen, and there is subintimal fibrosis in larger branches. This condition of hepatoportal sclerosis is accompanied by portal fibrosis and sometimes thrombosis[247].

Morphological diagnosis: *Arteries:* The diagnosis of arteriolosclerosis, polyarteriitis nodosa, and amyloidosis is made according to the usual criteria. *Veins:* Different stages of thrombosis with organization demand serial sections and staining for collagen fibers in addition to H & E. The same holds true for hepatoportal sclerosis and obliterative portal venopathy.

Differential diagnosis: Arterial lesions do not usually present major differential diagnostic problems. Amyloid may, however, be overlooked when there are only small amounts (p. 144).

Vein changes also give rise to few diagnostic problems. In many cases a liver cell carcinoma dominates the picture and the thrombosis may be overlooked.

Additional morphological findings: *Arteries:* Subintimal thickening may be seen in otherwise normal liver tissue and is usually not accompanied by any other specific changes.

In polyarteriitis nodosa orcein-positive ground glass cells can be demonstrated in a substantial number of patients[378]. Infarcts of the parenchyma have been described[51].

Amyloid in the artery wall may be found alone, but is virtually always accompanied by amyloid in the walls of the sinusoids[357]. *Veins:* As previously stated, thrombosis of the portal vein and its branches is most often seen in association with liver cell carcinoma[111a].

Schistosomal granulomas are often associated with portal fibrosis and thickened and tortuous veins. Schistosomal pigment may be found in Kupffer cells and portal macrophages[5].

Occurrence and significance: Thickening of the intima of the small arteries is seen in elderly patients and especially in those with hypertension. The polyarteritis nodosa lesion is part of a generalized connective tissue disease. When amyloid is present in portal vessles it is an expression of a generalized form. Thrombosis of portal vein branches must always raise suspicion of cirrhosis and liver cell carcinoma. However, non-cirrhotics may have so-called hepatoportal sclerosis[247]. Thrombi with a very high content of neutrophils are seen mainly in pyemic conditions[339].

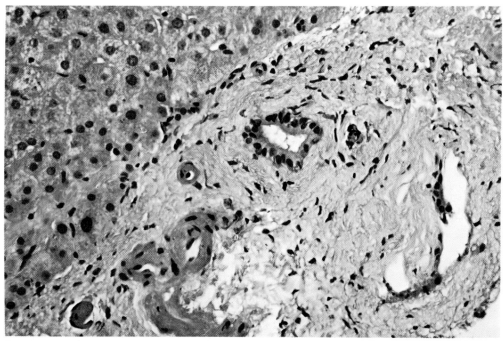

Fig. 48: Part of medium-sized portal tract with ramifications of a small artery showing transition to arterioles. A homogeneous eosinophil thickening of the intima is present. The patient had arterial hypertension (Needle biopsy, H & E x 270).

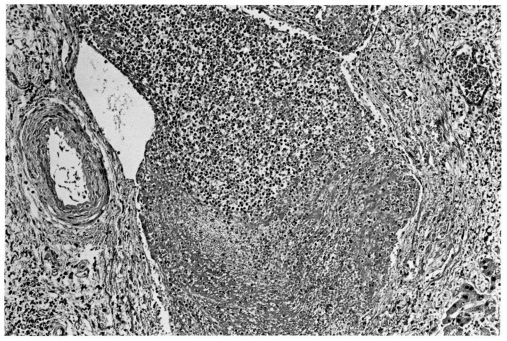

Fig. 49: Part of large portal tract with a large portal vein branch nearly completely filled by a thrombus dominated by fibrin in its lower part and neutrophils above (Autopsy, H & E x 110).

Malignant tumors

Morphology: The most common malignant tumor is metastatic carcinoma[136]. Less common are liver cell carcinoma, malignant lymphoma, leukemic infiltrations and cholangiocellular carcinoma.

Metastases may be of all sizes. All histological types occur but adenocarcinoma from the gastrointestinal tract (Fig. 50) and the breast and anaplastic carcinoma from the lung account for a large proportion[136]. Other examples are malignant melanoma, squamous cell carcinoma, choriocarcinoma, and leiomyosarcoma.

All forms of malignant lymphoma and leukemia may include the portal tracts of the liver and in most cases the parenchyma is also involved[4, 16, 145, 215]. The infiltrates in chronic lymphatic leukemia are better demarcated than those of other types of leukemia (Fig. 51).

Liver cell carcinoma in needle biopsies is generally found alone or together with cirrhotic liver tissue[84, 111d, 114, 254]. In most cases one or more portal tracts are invaded by tumor tissue.

Cholangiocellular carcinoma originates from portal bile ducts and early spread is in the portal tracts[111c].

Morphological diagnosis: The demonstration of malignant tumor tissue is as a rule easy since relatively large amounts are usually present. Small islands may, nevertheless, be overlooked unless multiple sections are performed. H & E-staining is useful as a routine but in special cases Alcian blue or staining for melanin is valuable. In malignant lymphoma and leukemia H & E may be supplemented by, e.g. PAS and methyl green pyronin.

Differential diagnosis: Metastatic carcinoma virtually never presents differential diagnostic difficulties with regard to the malignancy, although very well – differentiated adenocarcinomas from the pancreas may resemble proliferating bile ducts. Conversely, it may be difficult or impossible to decide whether an adenocarcinoma is primary or secondary, since primary adenocarcinomas represent a broad spectrum of histological variants[136] (p. 194).

Liver cell carcinomas can often be diagnosed as such, particularly when they are well or moderately differentiated. This is due to the similarity of the tumor cells to normal liver cells; of special significance is the presence of bile or Mallory bodies in the tumor cells[111d, 114]. Fat vacuoles, glycogen, globules and lipofuscin may also be demonstrable.

Malignant lymphomas and leukemic infiltrates also cause few differential diagnostic difficulties[4, 215]. Portal infiltrates in diffuse and nodular lymphomas may, however, sometimes resemble dense inflammatory infiltrates as seen in chronic persistent and chronic aggressive hepatitis. In hepatitis the inflammatory infiltrates comprise more different cell types, and the density of the infiltrates varies more than in lymphomas.

Additional morphological findings: Metastases are nearly always found in liver tissue with preserved lobular architecture[114]. In the parenchyma next to the tumor varying degrees of inflammation may be seen. Another common finding is parenchymal bile stasis and portal changes as found in large duct obstruction (p. 186). These changes are a virtually constant finding in cholangiocellular carcinoma[111c].

Liver cell carcinoma is most frequently associated with cirrhosis, in particular of macronodular pattern[254].

In malignant lymphoma and leukemia other changes in the liver are usually minimal and non-specific[4].

Occurrence and significance: Malignant tumor tissue is common in most series. Most common is metastatic adenocarcinoma. It is generally impossible to identify the primary site from histological appearance, and it may even be impossible, especially on poorly differentiated tumors, to distinguish between primary and secondary carcinoma[136]. Malignant melanoma, squamous cell carcinoma and choriocarcinoma are always metastatic.

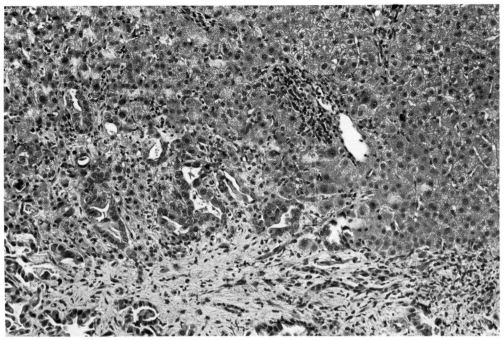

Fig. 50: Part of a large portal tract with irregularly distributed ductlike structures with some pleomorphism of the cells. A few similar structures are present in the adjacent parenchyma. Primary tumor in pancreas (Needle biopsy, H & E x 110).

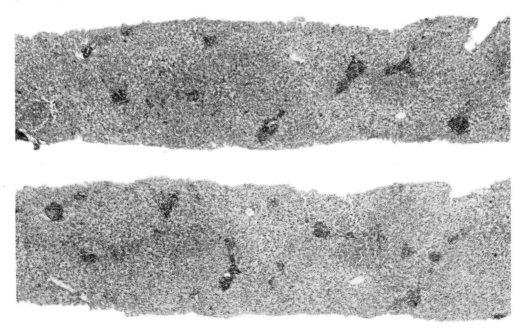

Fig. 51: Survey of a needle biopsy with slightly enlarged portal tracts with dense, uniform cellular infiltrations. The lobular architecture is well preserved and many normal central veins are seen. From a patient with chronic lymphatic leukemia (H & E x 30).

Normal

Morphology: The boundary between the portal tracts and the parenchyma is relatively sharp in normal liver tissue, and is composed of a plate-like structure, the limiting plate (syn.: lamina limitans). It comprises the layer of liver cells lying just beneath the connective tissue[11] (Fig. 52, see also Fig. 18 & 19).

Multiple small perforations of the limiting plate permit the passage of small bile ducts and of blood vessels; the latter are connected with the sinusoids[124].

The cells of the limiting plate are as a rule slightly smaller and more deeply stained than the rest of the liver cells[11]. These cells are in contact with sinusoids on one side only, while the cells of the internal liver plates are in contact with sinusoids on both sides.

The liver cells of the limiting plate often contain some lipofuscin granules. In relation to ramifications of the portal tree the limiting plate has normally an irregular outline (Fig. 53).

Morphological diagnosis: The histological recognition of normal limiting plates in a biopsy is usually easy. It is recommended to be made in low magnifications on sections stained with H & E and for collagen fibers.

Differential diagnosis: Portal inflammatory cells may infiltrate the limiting plate without con- comitant liver cell necrosis so-called spillover[94] (p. 34). In such cases the limiting plate is preserved.

Sometimes a newly formed, dislocated limiting plate may be mistaken for a normal one. Staining for collagen fibers in many cases permits differentiation between the mature connective tissue of the original portal tract and the younger, more loosely structured connective tissue constituting the periportal fibrosis[94] (p. 158).

Additional morphological findings: If all the limiting plates in a biopsy are normal, other changes are often absent, but in many cases of steatosis, siderosis, "pure" cholestasis and even acute hepatitis a normal lamina limitans may be found.

Occurrence and significance: The diagnostic significance of a preserved and normal lamina limitans is due to the fact that a long list of diagnoses can be excluded, provided that many portal tracts with preserved lamina limitans are represented in the biopsy. Examples are chronic aggressive hepatitis and cirrhosis. In the earlier stages of large duct obstruction the limiting plate is usually preserved, but if the condition persists for more than 2 to 3 weeks, destruction is usual[138, 327e].

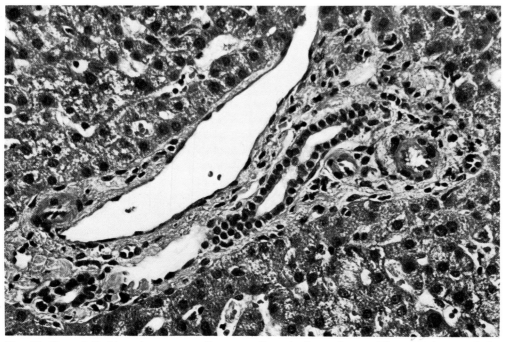

Fig. 52: Normal limiting plate surrounding a medium-sized portal tract. The plate is smooth in relation to the upper left and lower borders of the tract but slightly irregular in the upper right area (Needle biopsy, H & E x 270).

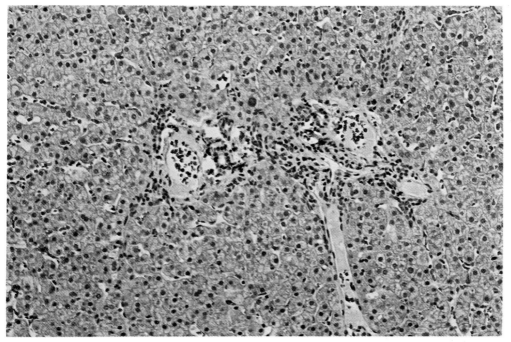

Fig. 53: Two normal portal tracts with many ramifications, mainly the right. The limiting plates are correspondingly somewhat irregular but normal (Needle biopsy, H & E x 110).

Destruction

Morphology: The limiting plate or part of it is destroyed as a result of necrosis of a varying number of the liver cells constituting the plate. Small lesions may be found as part of focal liver cell necrosis widely distributed in the lobules. Necrosis may also be selective and affect the limiting plate. Such necrosis is seen in two forms. The first is so-called piecemeal necrosis[29, 31, 89] which is to be found as smaller or larger wedgeshaped lesions accompanied by a dense infiltrate dominated by lymphocytes and plasma cells. The second form is present together with marginal bile duct proliferation and edema of the portal connective tissue; these changes are initially small, and surrounded by an infiltrate composed mainly of neutrophils[67, 138, 291] (Fig. 54).

When the necroses are small, the defects are as a rule replaced by newly formed liver cells, and normal conditions are reestablished. When the defects are larger, and especially when the processes progress and destroy the reticulin framework, new connective tissue is formed from the portal tracts with deposition of collagen fibers and splitting up of the peripheral parts of the lobules (periportal fibrosis)[31, 94] (Fig. 55). One may consequently see defects of the limiting plate filled by liver cell remnants (with inflammation) or connective tissue, or both[31, 94].

With further progression of the necrosis and fibrosis the splitting of the parenchyma may involve whole lobules. However, when the processes cease after having involved the peripheral parts of the lobules only, new limiting plates are formed at a distance from the margins of the portal tracts[94].

Morphological diagnosis: Recognition of a partly or completely destroyed limiting plate is easiest in sections stained for collagen fibers (or, less reliably, reticulin fibers) and can be achieved at low magnifications. It is important at the same time to register whether the defects contain necrotic liver cell material or whether there is new connective tissue.

Differential diagnosis: As indicated above, destruction of the limiting plate is usually easy to recognize. Mild degrees may be confused, however, with so-called spillover[94] (p. 34). Furthermore, a dislocated limiting plate may be mistaken for a normal one[94]. Staining for collagen fibers, preferably van Gieson staining, helps to distinguish between the original mature portal connective tissue and the more weakly stained connective tissue comprising the periportal fibrosis. Not until 6–12 months and usually only after several years do the differences grow indistinct.

Additional morphological findings: Destruction of the limiting plate by piecemeal necrosis is most characteristically seen in chronic aggressive hepatitis[31, 89] and in some cases of acute hepatitis[29, 31]. Similar findings may also be observed in primary biliary cirrhosis[93, 325] and Wilson's disease[205, 323]. Necroses with many neutrophils are typically seen in large duct obstruction[67, 138].

Pronounced fibrosis of the limiting plate and the adjacent parts of the parenchyma is a prerequisite for the diagnosis of chronic aggressive hepatitis[31, 89]. Slight fibrosis of the limiting plate is a common finding in the late stages of acute hepatitis[29, 31] and may also be seen in chronic persistent hepatitis[89].

Occurrence and significance: Slight destruction of the limiting plate as part of focal liver cell necrosis is recorded in a large proportion of all cases of acute hepatitis and has no prognostic implications[265]. On the other hand most cases with larger defects due to piecemeal necrosis progress to chronic aggressive hepatitis[101]. Similarly most of the cases of chronic aggressive hepatitis with many and large defects of the limiting plate have a great tendency to develop cirrhosis[99].

The destruction of the limiting plate seen in large duct obstruction is most often focal and does not extend far into the lobules[67, 138]. When the obstruction persists, however, splitting up of the lobules may occur and cirrhosis develop (secondary biliary cirrhosis)[327f].

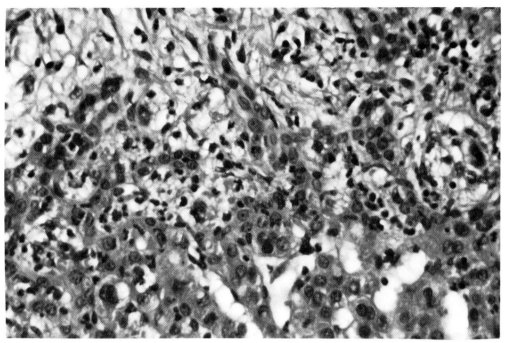

Fig. 54: Peripheral area of a medium-sized portal tract. The limiting plate is destroyed and in its place debris, inflammation, edema and proliferating bile ducts are found. From a patient with large duct obstruction (Surgical biopsy, H & E x 270).

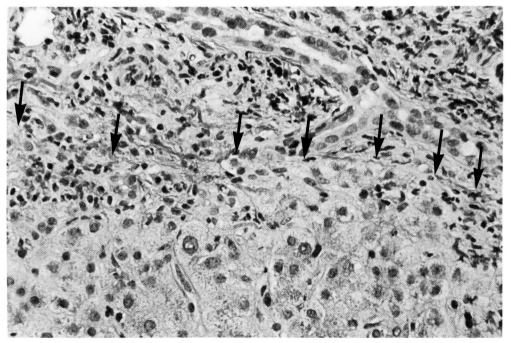

Fig. 55: Peripheral part of a large portal tract. The limiting plate is destroyed and its original location indicated by arrows. Marginal bile duct proliferation and inflammation are seen. Large duct obstruction for 3 months (Surgical biopsy, van Gieson x 270).

Normal

Morphology: Three-dimensional reconstructions of normal liver tissue make it probable that the liver cells are arranged in anastomosing plates – a so-called muralium – surrounded by sinusoids[124]. In the newborn the plates are two to three liver cells thick, but from the age of 3 to 6 they are only one cell thick[241]. The plates are in many locations perforated by communications between the sinusoids. Each liver cell is thus in larger children and adults contiguous with the sinusoids on at least two facets.

The lining cells of the sinusoids are separated slightly from the liver cell plates by the space of Disse[81]. Normally this space cannot be seen with the light microscope[269]. It contains, however, a fine network of supporting reticulin fibers and in sections stained for these fibers one can see the many and fine, mainly longitudinally running threads. Such sections give a very clear impression of the thickness of the liver cell plates and their radial arrangement around the central vein. The plates can, except where perforated by sinusoids, be followed from the portal tracts to the central veins, and they are normally nearly straight and without significant variation in thickness.

Four to nine facets of the liver cell surface are in contact with neighboring liver cells, and these facets contain grooves which delimit bile canaliculi[35, 82]. The part of the cell membrane which forms the wall of the canaliculi project irregularly into the lumen as short microvilli. The membranes of either side of the lumen are tightly bound together by a junctional complex. In some cases the bile canaliculus bifurcates to form two or three long branches running on the same facet of the cell, but as a rule only a single channel runs between each adjacent pair of cells. Thus the bile canaliculi form a network having mainly hexagonal meshes in the plate, and three dimensionally they form an anastomosing net with polyhedral meshes. The bile drains in general in the direction of the periphery of the lobule, where it enters into small bile ducts.

Morphological diagnosis: The identification of normal liver cell plates is made in sections stained with H & E and for reticulin fibers (Fig. 56 & 57). To be diagnosed as normal the plates must not only be of normal thickness but also have a normal orientation with radial arrangement around the central veins, and abutting on the portal tracts at right angles. Bile canaliculi are normally not seen and do not contain visible bile. The canaliculi can be demonstrated by staining for alkaline phosphatases[358].

Differential diagnosis: The recognition of normal liver cell plates is relatively easy. Slighter degrees of, e.g. centrilobular variation in liver-cell size resulting in a slight variation of the plate thickness may, however, be overlooked. Such a slight, mainly centrilobular irregularity is characteristic for the late stage of acute hepatitis[29] (p. 172).

An apparently normal extent of liver cell plates of normal thickness may be found in areas of larger parenchymal nodules in macronodular cirrhosis[7]. Such areas are usually of limited size and multiple sections are of great importance.

Additional morphological findings: When all the liver cell plates in a biopsy are normal, the liver tissue is as a rule normal. Slight changes such as mild steatosis or mild non-specific reactive hepatitis may, however, be present. On the other hand liver tissue in severe diseases such as chronic aggressive hepatitis and cirrhosis may include areas with normal appering plates.

Occurence and significance: A small but significant part of our biopsy material consists of liver tissue with normal plates, either in entirely normal liver or combined with modest changes such as mild degrees of steatosis or non-specific hepatitis.

A complete lack of normal plates is virtually always tantamount to severe liver damage, e.g. severe forms of acute hepatitis or active phases of chronic aggressive hepatitis or cirrhosis.

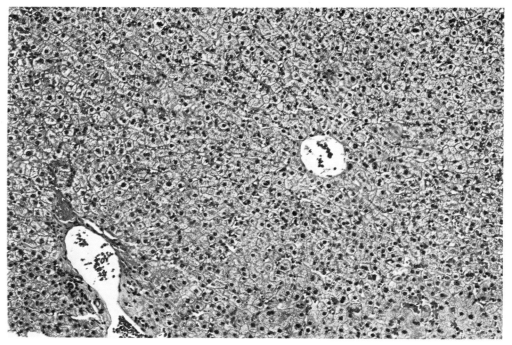

Fig. 56: Part of normal liver lobule with a portal tract (lower left) and a central vein. The liver cell plates are inconspicuous in many areas (Needle biopsy, H & E x 110).

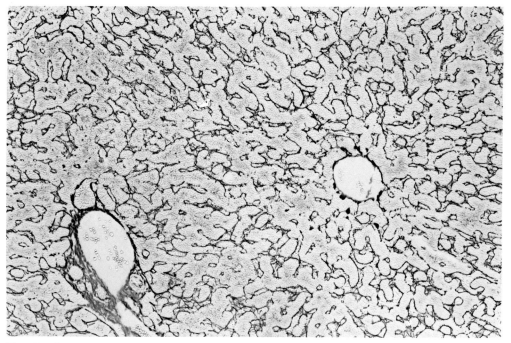

Fig. 57: Same areas as shown above. The section is stained for reticulin fibers illustrating the demarcation of the liver cell plates which radiate from the central vein (Needle biopsy, reticulin x 110).

Abnormal thickness

Morphology: In livers with preserved lobular architecture one may find the plates narrowed or thickened.

Narrowed plates are associated either with sinusoidal dilatation or with deposits of amyloid in the space of Disse.

In sinusoidal dilatation, which is nearly always centrilobular or mainly centrilobular, varying degrees of liver cell atrophy are demonstrable[295]. This results in a corresponding narrowing of the plates (Fig. 58). Similar changes may be seen either in the periportal or in the intermediate zones[395]. The liver cells are smaller than normal and narrowed between the sinusoids, and often show increased eosinophilia of the cytoplasm.

In exceptional cases such as peliosis there is subtotal or complete atrophy of parts of the liver cell plates[399].

Amyloid is located primarily in the space of Disse and is seen as homogeneous, eosinophilic material in H & E-stained sections (p. 144). The amyloid is associated with both atrophy of the liver cell plates and narrowing of the sinusoids[357].

Thickened plates are either caused by an increased number of cells or by enlarged, edematous liver cells, so-called ballooning. When the number of cells is increased, the plates are most often two cells thick, but may contain three or even more (Fig. 59). The liver cells are usually smaller and with more basophilic cytoplasm than normal. These changes may involve whole lobules, but are most commonly found in the intermediate and the periportal zone.

When the thickening of the plates is caused by ballooning of the liver cells, this is most often predominantly centrilobular and associated with focal changes such as necrosis of the cells and collapse of the plates; the result is centrilobular plates which vary more in thickness than normal.

Morphological diagnosis: Deviation of the caliber of the liver cell plates from normal is best identified in sections stained for reticulin fibers in combination with H & E-stained sections (Fig. 59).

Slight atrophy or slight thickening may be difficult to recognize and serial sections may be valuable. The diagnosis is supported when the distribution is zonal.

Differential diagnosis: Artefacts produced by fixation and seen in a narrow zone along the margin of the biopsy may cause differential diagnostic problems[212]. Most often the plates are narrowed but may vary in thickness. The most important feature is that the artefacts are localized to the marginal parts of the biopsy and have no zonal distribution.

Additional morphological findings: In addition to centrilobular atrophy of the plates and dilatation of the sinusoids, one often finds steatosis in the intermediate or periportal zones, and sometimes confluent centrilobular necrosis[73, 390] (p. 86). Cholestasis is common in severe cases, and in prolonged disease fibrosis may develop[73, 342].

Thickened plates and plates of varying thickness are most common in acute viral hepatitis (p. 172). Amyloid deposits can in most cases be demonstrated also in portal vessels (p. 60).

Occurrence and significance: Centrilobular atrophy and sinusoidal dilatation is above all found in venous congestion caused by right-sided heart failure[37, 295, 342]. For other causes, see p. 198.

Thickened plates with an increased number of liver cells are an expression of a high rate of regeneration and are usually seen after extensive liver cell necrosis, for example in acute hepatitis or after cardiac shock[338]. The presence of areas with thickened plates suggests incipient restitution.

Plates of varying thickness are usually due to a mixture of retrograde and regenerative liver cell changes. They are most characteristically seen in acute hepatitis and have diagnostic importance[265, 289].

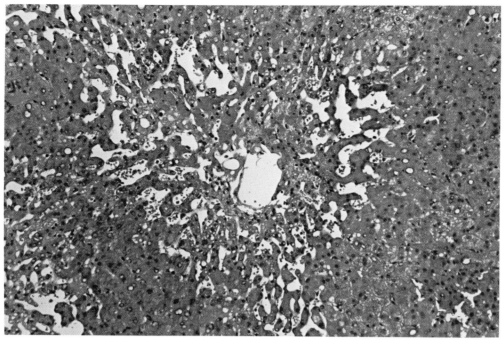

Fig. 58: Part of lobule with central vein in the center. A pronounced centrilobular and intermediary sinusoidal dilatation with accompanying atrophy of the liver cell plates is demonstrated. From a patient with right-sided heart failure (Needle biopsy, H & E x 110).

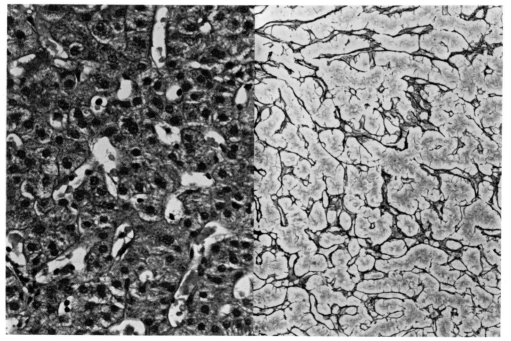

Fig. 59: Left. Thickened liver cell plates often two to three cells thick (H & E). Right. Same biopsy (reticulin). From a patient in the recovery period after a severe acute hepatitis with extended panlobular necrosis (Surgical biopsy x 270).

Abnormal configuration

Morphology: In livers with preserved lobular architecture the liver cells may under certain circumstances be arranged in rounded or abnormal longitudinal formations. Three-dimensional reconstructions have shown that the structures are spherical, ovoid or cylindrical and consist of a single cell layer surrounding a central lumen[258]. In this lumen a bile thrombus is commonly present, and histochemical and ultrastructural investigations have indicated that the lumen is probably delimited by the biliary poles of the liver cells. The spherical and ovoid structures are called *rosettes* (syn. pseudoacini or adenomatous proliferation) (Fig. 60) and the cylindrical ones are named *tubules* (syn. pseudoglandular proliferation) (Fig. 61). The formation of these lesions imitates the architecture of the liver of some low vertebrates, in which the organ is a ramified, tubular gland[23].

Rosettes may be circular or oval depending on the plane of section. They are encircled by a network of reticulin fibers. The liver cells which form part of the lesions, sometimes appear normal under the light microscope, but are often altered. They are either ballooned or they are small with basophilic cytoplasm, sometimes with more than one nucleus. The smallest rosettes comprise only three cells, and the lumen may be difficult to recognize. In most cases a conspicuous lumen with or without bile thrombus is, however, present. Around the rosettes one often finds cellular debris from liver cell necrosis and inflammatory cells.

Tubules have a rounded form when cut at right angles, but as a rule a substantial proportion are cut more or less longitudinally and are consequently tubular[350]. Both form and extent vary.

Morphological diagnosis: Abundant and conspicuous rosettes are easily identified even at low magnifications. Few and small rosettes are, on the other hand, only diagnosed after careful search at higher magnifications. It is recommended that conventional sections and sections stained for reticulin fibers be used.

Tubules are usually recognized even at low magnification.

Differential diagnosis: The lesions in question have a very characteristic appearance and they do not cause differential diagnostic difficulties.

Additional morphological findings: Rosettes are common in severe forms of acute hepatitis[245, 348] and chronic aggressive hepatitis[93] and are most often seen in close relation to liver cell necrosis and inflammation.

In so-called "pure" cholestasis it is usually possible to find some rosettes, and in some instances there are many[30]. In early stages the rosettes are devoid of visible necrosis and inflammation, and the liver cells are of normal size and stainability. Later necrosis, inflammation and some ballooning of the liver cells may develop.

In early large duct obstruction the lobules are similarly without other changes apart from cholestasis (p. 186).

Occurrence and significance: Rosettes are common in ordinary biopsy material. They are essentially seen in conditions with extensive liver cell necrosis, e.g. severe cases of acute hepatitis and chronic aggressive hepatitis, and the lesion is then probably an expression of regeneration[245]. In liver tissue with preserved lobular architecture the rosette is a temporary lesion, and the liver may return to normal when the necrosis and cholestasis disappear.

Tubules are characteristically seen in a series of congenital disturbances of carbohydrate or protein metabolism. Good examples are galactosamia[350], tyrosinosis[201] and fructose intolerance[141]. It is probable that the formation of tubules in these cases is genetically determined.

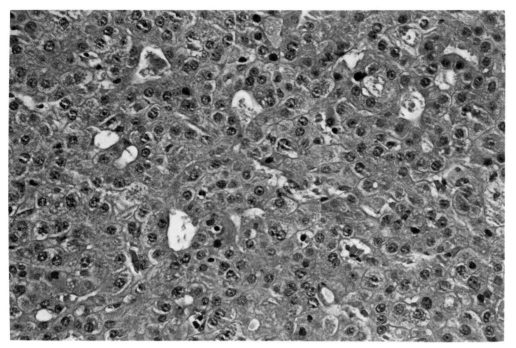

Fig. 60: Multiple liver cell rosettes from a patient with pure cholestasis following testosterone. The lumina are dilated and often contain eosinophilic material. In other parts of the biopsy (not demonstrated) cholestasis is conspicuous (Needle biopsy, H & E x 270).

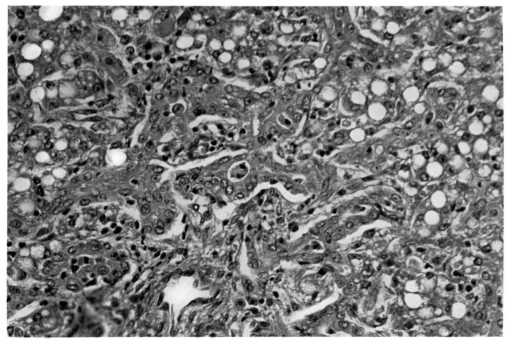

Fig. 61: Portal tract and periportal part of the parenchyma showing marked tubular proliferation. Many of the cells in the tubules have features of bile duct epithelium while others look similar to liver cells (galactosemia) (Autopsy specimen, H & E x 270).

Abnormal in parenchymal nodules

Morphology: The parenchymal nodules are composed of liver cells arranged in irregular, often partly anastomosing liver cell plates, most often one to two cells thick and of different length (Fig. 62 & 63). In between the irregularly arranged plates in the nodules there are as a rule sinusoids, but areas with capillaries, often with dense collagen fibers in their wall may be found, or elsewhere, hyalinized connective tissue with only few vessels[7].

Narrowed plates occur, as in liver tissue with preserved lobular architecture, in association with sinusoidal dilatation[295] or with deposits of amyloid[357]. The liver cells are smaller than normal, narrowed and often with slightly increased eosinophilia of the cytoplasm.

Occasionally one may find smaller or larger areas of parenchymal nodules composed of newly formed liver cell plates with small cells, basophilic cytoplasm, "active" nuclei, cells with two or three nuclei, and possibly mitoses. These cells may show all transitions to dysplasia[7, 274], and it is probable that such areas may represent points of origin for liver cell carcinoma. Thickening of the liver cell plates in parenchymal nodules is often caused by an increase in the number of cells. The thickened plates are most often two cells thick but there may be more. As a rule one finds areas of such plates in most nodules.

What has been said about rosettes and tubules in liver tissue with preserved lobular architecture (p. 72) also holds true in livers with parenchymal nodules. In this context it should be noted that both rosettes and tubules can also be found in certain histological types of liver cell adenoma[19, 189] and liver cell carcinoma[84, 111d, 114].

Morphological diagnosis: Abnormally thick liver cell plates in parenchymal nodules are easily recognized in routine stainings. Rosettes may be difficult to identify, and their diagnosis usually demands a careful search of the sections at higher magnifications.

Differential diagnosis: When changes are minimal or doubtful, serial sections are necessary. In most other cases no differential diagnostic problems exist.

Additional morphological findings: Abnormal liver cell plates in parenchymal nodules are found in cirrhosis, and all the other changes described in relation to cirrhosis may be found. Rosettes occur most often in cirrhosis with pronounced activity and with regeneration of the liver cells. Cholestasis is commonly found in the lumens. Thickened liver cell plates in parenchymal nodules are also seen in nodular regenerative hyperplasia[360] (p. 26).

Occurrence and significance: The presence of irregularly orientated liver cell plates of varying thickness is of diagnostic value for the diagnosis of cirrhosis, especially in fragmented biopsies from a macronodular pattern of disease. It must be stressed, however, that multilayered and irregular plates can only give rise to a suspicion of cirrhosis, and a firm diagnosis requires the demonstration of nodules with fibrosis[7].

Changes in the morphology of the liver cell plates in cirrhosis arise in periods of destruction and attempted regeneration[274]. The thickening of liver cell plates is an expression of increased liver cell proliferation and mainly follows extensive liver cell necrosis, but in some cases the above-mentioned new formation of basophilic liver cells may apparently, occur without preceding necrosis. This type of proliferation may be an early sign of malignant transformation[7, 274].

Atrophy of the plates is in cirrhosis a more or less local phenomenon without characteristic localization. Sinusoidal dilatation with atrophy may result from cardiac insufficiency in patients with cirrhosis as well as in those with previously normal livers.

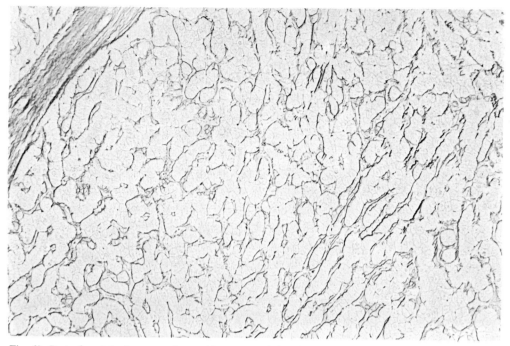

Fig. 62: Part of nodule from a patient with macronodular cirrhosis. The plates are of varying breath and length, partly anastomosing and irregularly orientated (Needle biopsy, reticulin x 110).

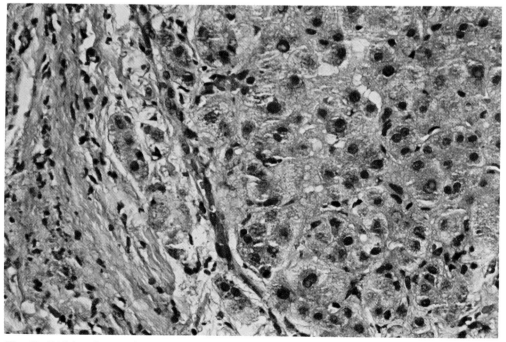

Fig. 63: Peripheral part of a nodule, from a patient with posthepatitic cirrhosis. Some of the liver cells are small and crowded with dark nuclei. They are arranged in thick plates with some characteristic rosettes ("regeneration zone") (Needle biopsy, H & E x 270).

Cholestasis

Morphology: Morphological cholestasis is defined as bile pigment in sections visible under the light microscope[67, 92, 95, 293] (Fig. 64 & 65). The cholestasis is most often seen as so-called bile thrombi situated in dilated canaliculi. The thrombi may have all sizes, from hardly visible to several microns. The shape varies from circular to more or less longitudinal structures, the latter often v- og y-shaped. Bile pigment can in addition be found in liver cells, in histiocytes both in parenchyma and in portal tracts, and in portal bile ducts. In the liver cells and in the histiocytes the pigment is found as small thrombi or as granules.

The color of the thrombi depends on several factors[92, 95]. The larger the thrombus, the darker the color. In early cholestasis the color is usually greenish, whereas later often it becomes more brown.

Cholestasis can be found in all degrees from a single, small thrombus in a biopsy to numerous and large thrombi, and it is characteristic that cholestasis in the early stages is centrilobular, while longer – lasting conditions are associated with a more widespread and often mainly periportal location[92, 293]. In cirrhosis the cholestasis is as a rule without characteristic localization.

Morphological diagnosis: In severe cholestasis the biopsy is green on naked eye inspection, and the number of bile thrombi is so high and their size so big that the diagnosis can be made even at low magnification. Small bile thrombi may, however, be missed. They are best demonstrated at high magnification in sections stained for iron or with van Gieson. The green color is particularly bright in the latter (Fig. 65).

Differential diagnosis: Bile thrombi almost never give differential diagnostic problems when sections stained for iron or with van Gieson are used. Only typical green deposits are diagnostic. Small clumps may be difficult to distinguish from lipofuscin, ceroid or Dubin-Johnson pigment in H & E[92]. Special stains are helpful (p. 122).

Pigment in erythropoietic protoporphyria resembles bile[83]. Polarization microscopy provides specific identification.

Additional morphological findings: Centrilobular cholestasis, by far the most common form, is usually an expression of short duration and is in particular seen in large duct obstruction[138, 291] (p. 186), acute hepatitis[29, 265] (p. 174) and in liver lesions following drugs[30, 187, 272] (p. 184).

Periportal cholestasis is characteristic of a long duration and is especially found in large duct obstruction[67, 138, 291] and in primary biliary cirrhosis[279, 325], but may also be seen in a few cases of chronic aggressive hepatitis[58, 89].

In cirrhosis the cholestasis is as a rule most pronounced in the secondary biliary form[327f] and in the late stages of primary biliary cirrhosis[325]. Severe cholestasis may in addition be met with in both alcoholic and posthepatitic cirrhosis; the cholestasis is then usually more focal than is the case in the biliary forms[274].

Occurrence and significance: Morphological cholestasis is as a rule found in patients with jaundice but the agreement between clinical and morphologic findings is not complete[95]. Thus bile thrombi may be found in relation to focal lesions, e.g. tumors, in non-icteric patients, and conversely, morphologic cholestasis is sometimes absent from biopsies from jaundiced patients. The latter phemonenon may at least partly be explained by washing out of smaller bile thrombi during the technical procedures[95]. Bile thrombi persist in a few cases for weeks after the disappearance of jaundice, and the rule is that the bile pigment in histiocytes comes and goes later than in canaliculi and liver cells.

Liver biopsies in a substantial number of cases permit distinction between intra- and extrapehatic cholestasis[293] (p. 186). This is especially so in "pure" cholestasis (p. 184) and in cholestasis in typical acute hepatitis (p. 174).

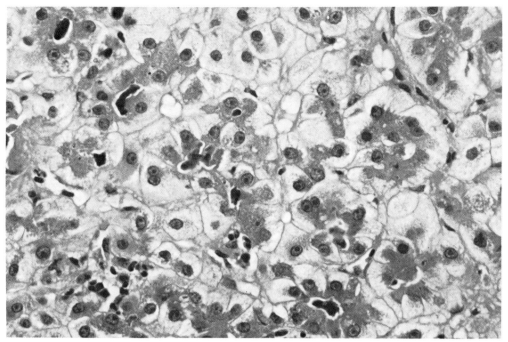

Fig. 64: Part of liver lobule with several bile thrombi. Some are black while others are orange. All the thrombi are found in relation to rosettes. From a patient with acute viral hepatitis (Needle biopsy, H & E x 270).

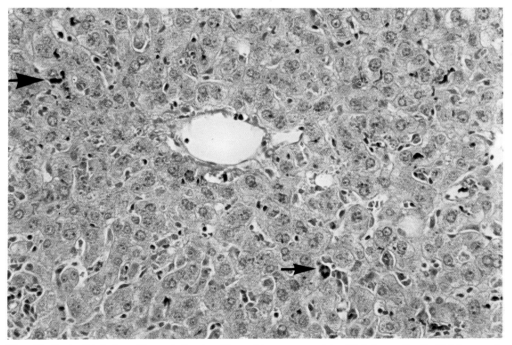

Fig. 65: Part of lobule with central vein. Thrombi are present in dilated canaliculi (thick arrow) and in Kupffer cells (thin arrow). From a case of jaundice after 14-ketosteroid treatment (Needle biopsy, van Gieson x 270).

Normal

Morphology: Human liver cells or hepatocytes appear three-dimensionally in three basic shapes as penta-, octa- or decahedrons, their shape and size depending on their position in the muralium[120]. Cells occupying corners where plates meet are usually larger, while cells in the middle of the walls are generally smaller. The smallest cells are often found surrounding perforations in the liver plates. This dependence of the volume of the liver cells on their location is also evident in two-dimensional histological sections, in which the liver cells are polygonal with distinct boundaries[119, 120].

The liver cell nucleus is round to ovoid with a well-defined nuclear membrane and one or more nucleoli. The number and size of nuclei per cell are most probably determined by the volume of the cell, and the larger cells contain either two or more nuclei or one diploid or tetraploid nucleus so that the total mass of chromatin is adequate for the volume of cytoplasm[72, 214], Mitoses are rare.

The liver cell has three physiological surfaces. Two or three facets are in contact with the space of Disse. These facets are often called the "vascular pole"[120]. Four to nine facets are in contact with neighboring liver cells, and these facets contain several grooves which delimit canaliculi. These grooves are often called the "biliary pole"[120].

On the facets where the cells are in contact with the space of Disse the cell membranes project into the space in the form of numerous microvilli[49, 130]. Normally neither bile canaliculi nor the space of Disse can be seen with the light microscope. The cytoplasm of the liver cells is faintly eosinophilic in H & E-stained sections with many minute, diffusely distributed basophilic granules. The normal liver cell always contains glycogen, but the amount varies partly according to a diurnal rythm and partly according to the localization in the lobule[91, 321]. Furthermore some glycogen is washed out during histological preparation. Glycogen can be demonstrated by PAS-staining. The normal liver cells do not contain fat or iron[321], but virtually always – except in infants and children – lipo-

fuscin which in H & E-stained sections is seen as golden-brown, fine granules. Under normal circumstances most lipofuscin is found in the liver cells in the centrilobular area (Fig. 139).

Morphological diagnosis: It is usually easy to determine whether liver cells are normal or pathological (Fig. 66 & 67). The recognition of small changes in size of both cells and nuclei may be difficult – because of the above-mentioned normal variation – and demands some experience. The presence of fat, Mallory bodies, bile or iron in the cytoplasm excludes the diagnosis of normal liver cells. The same holds true when rosettes or abnormal plates are present. H & E is the most important staining method, but since, for instance small amounts of copper and iron are very diffucult or impossible to recognize with this stain, it is always helpful to supplement H & E with appropriate special stains.

Differential diagnosis: The recognition of normal liver cells is usually easy, but one must always keep in mind that the omission of different special staining procedures reduces the certainty with which abnormalities can be excluded.

Additional morphological findings: When all liver cells in a biopsy are normal, the biopsy itself is probably from normal liver. It must be remembered, however, that areas with normal appearing liver cells may be found in many conditions and even in diseases such as acute and chronic hepatitis, drug reactions, and cirrhosis.

Occurrence and significance: Biopsies in which all liver cells are normal account for only a small percentage in most series. Such livers are most often normal but in the early stages of so-called "pure" cholestasis the liver cells also appear normal[30]. It should furthermore be remembered that normal or virtually normal liver cells may be found in some cases of chronic persistent hepatitis[89].

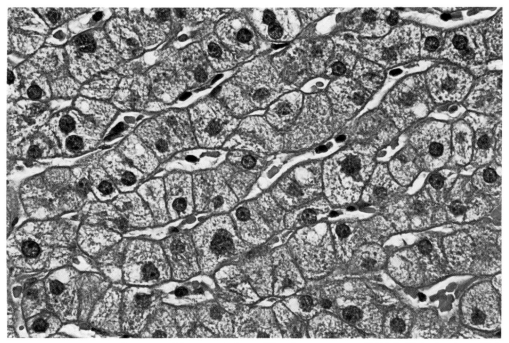

Fig. 66: Normal liver cells arranged in normal plates. The plates are one cell thick. Note the sinusoidal lining cells and the erythrocytes in some of the sinusoids (Needle biopsy, H & E x 400).

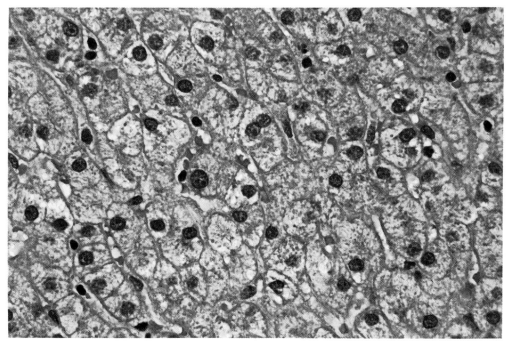

Fig. 67: Another biopsy from a normal liver. This specimen is less well fixated than the specimen above and some details are lost. (Needle biopsy, H & E x 400).

Acidophil bodies

Morphology: Acidophil bodies are roundish bodies of the size of or smaller than normal liver cells[184, 273, 316]. They are pushed out of the liver cell plates, often surrounded by a clear slit, and, as a rule, without special relation to inflammatory cells. An acidophil body is a changed liver cell and appears well demarcated. It is strongly eosinophilic, and the structure is homogeneous, although in many cases one may see a pyknotic nucleus or nuclear debris (Fig. 68). Sometimes the condensed cytoplasm contains some lipofuscin granules and in a few cases fat droplets or bile thrombi.

The acidophil body is a special form of single cell necrosis called shrinkage necrosis or apoptosis[316, 317, 321]. This form of necrosis is claimed to be an active, inherently programmed, phenomenon, which is also seen under physiological conditions. No cell breakdown products are released into the surrounding tissue and therefore inflammatory cells are seldom seen. The changes comprise a condensation and clumping of the cell nucleus and to some degree also of the cytoplasm. The mitochondria remain both structurally and probably also functionally uninjured for some time[191, 317]. The shrinkage processes continue slowly, and fragmentation gradually takes place. The fragments are phagocytosed by histiocytes and Kupffer cells[273, 316].

Acidophil bodies occur in all areas of the lobules. In the early stages of acute hepatitis most are found, however, in the centrilobular and intermediary zone[265, 317].

Morphological diagnosis: Acidophil bodies may easily be missed at smaller magnification. Demonstration is preferably made at 2–300 x magnification on H & E-stained sections and is primarily based on the roundish form, the eosinophilic staining and their presence outside the liver cell plates.

Differential diagnosis: Histiocytes and Kupffer cells which have phagocytosed abundant material may have a rounded form. However, their nuclei are well preserved and the cytoplasm is virtually never homogeneous or strongly eosinophilic, and these cells are not separated from the liver cell plates by a slit.

Additional morphological findings: A limited number of acidophil bodies may be found in a great variety of conditions (Fig. 69), and one may see one or a few even in otherwise normal liver biopsy material[53]. A large number are characteristically present in acute hepatitis[29, 265], but there may also be many in active forms of cirrhosis[63] and chronic aggressive hepatitis[58]. They are similar to the so-called Councilman bodies in yellow fever[53].

Occurrence and significance: As indicated above, one or a few acidophil bodies may be found in otherwise normal liver tissue, and the demonstration of a few dispersed bodies therefore has no diagnostic significance[53]. The presence of many bodies shows, however, that liver damage is taking place[273, 316]. In our experience many acidophil bodies are a constant feature of acute hepatitis[265] and acidophil bodies are consequently a prerequisite for this diagnosis[29, 265].

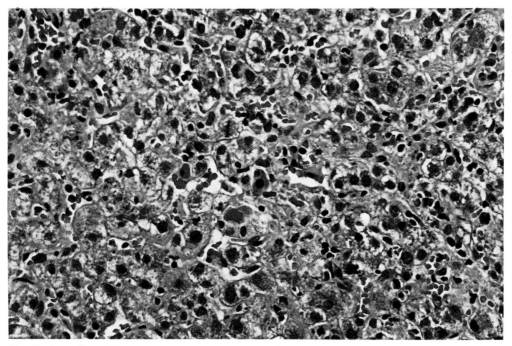

Fig. 68: Part of a lobule with acidophil bodies some of which contain pyknotic nuclear material and some of which are without nuclear remnants. From a case of acute viral hepatitis (Needle biopsy, H & E x 270).

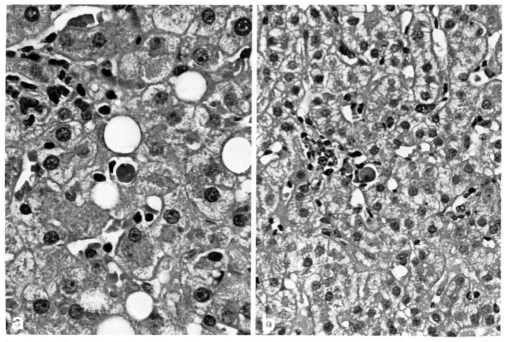

Fig. 69: Left. Acidophil body in a biopsy showing slight to moderate steatosis. Right. Acidophil body in a biopsy with only minimal changes of the nonspecific reactive hepatitis type (Needle biopsies, H & E left x 400, right x 270).

Focal with Kupffer cell proliferation

Morphology: Focal liver cell necrosis is a lytic necrosis seen as defects of the liver cell plates involving single cells or small groups of cells[273, 327a] (Fig. 70 & 71). Following rupture of the membrane the cell content is expelled and the cell outline is no longer visible, and therefore focal or spotty necrosis is often best recognized by the accumulation of inflammatory cells replacing the necrotic hepatocytes. The inflammatory reaction is usually composed of histiocytes, lymphocytes, plasma cells, and hypertrophied Kupffer cells, and it is this type of focal necrosis which will be described in the following paragraphs. However, the inflammatory reaction is occasionally dominated by neutrophils[70] (p. 96). Focal necrosis occurs in all areas of the lobules but is sometimes most pronounced in the centrilobular area.

Morphological diagnosis: Focal liver cell necrosis can in most cases be identified at smaller magnification in H & E-stained sections. Very small defects of the liver cell plates filled with histiocytes and Kupffer cells may be overlooked and higher magnifications are recommended.

Differential diagnosis: Accumulation of inflammatory cells in the sinusoids, and focal Kupffer cell proliferation – both without necrosis – may look similar to focal liver cell necrosis, but in these cases no defects in the liver cell plates are demonstrable.

Tangentially cut lipogranulomas may also have an appearance very similar to focal liver cell necrosis, but the macrophages in the lipogranulomas have the character of lipophages and – by using serial sections – one can nearly always demonstrate a central fat vacuole[57].

Additional morphological findings: Focal liver cell necrosis occurs in varying degrees together with many different parenchymal and portal changes. Even in biopsies without pathological changes one or a few small dispersed areas of necrosis may be found[327a]. In these cases the rest of the hepatocytes appear normal, and the histiocytes contain little or no ceroid.

Severe, mainly centrilobular focal necrosis is characteristic for acute hepatitis[29, 31, 265]. The histiocytes typically contain abundant PAS-positive, diastase – resistant material and the surrounding liver cells are often ballooned.

Occurrence and significance: Slight focal necrosis is of no diagnostic significance[327a]. Severe, rounded mainly centrilobular focal liver cell necrosis is strongly suggestive of acute hepatitis, and it can be said that focal necrosis of this type is a *conditio sine qua non* for this histological diagnosis[29, 31, 265]. In this context it must also be mentioned that a similar histological picture is to be found in some cases of drug-induced liver damage.

Severe focal liver cell necrosis may also be demonstrated in cases of active cirrhosis[63] and chronic aggressive hepatitis[58].

Focal necrosis with Kupffer cell proliferation is in addition to be found in non-specific reactive hepatitis (p. 180). Usually the lesion has a more irregular form than in acute hepatitis.

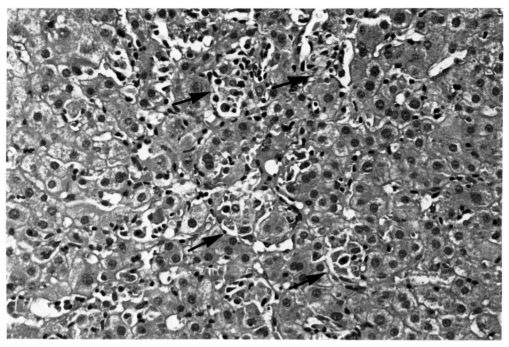

Fig. 70: Part of a lobule demonstrating multiple lesions of focal liver cell necrosis; some of the focal lesions are indicated by arrows. In addition an acidophil body is seen (lower left quadrant). Acute viral hepatitis (Needle biopsy, H & E x 270).

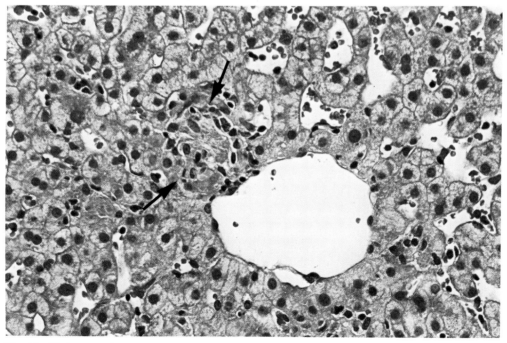

Fig. 71: High magnification of a focal liver cell necrosis demarcated by arrows. In the area of necrosis cell debris, lymphocytes and histiocytes are found. The lesion is located close to a central vein. Acute viral hepatitis (Needle biopsy, H & E x 400).

Piecemeal

Morphology: Piecemeal necrosis is necrosis of liver cells at a parenchymal-connective tissue interface accompanied by infiltration with lymphocytes and plasma cells[58, 89, 278, 327a] (Fig. 72 & 73). In livers with preserved lobular architecture it is to be found in the periportal zone, associated with destruction of the limiting plate, or in relation to fibrous septa. In cirrhosis it is seen in the peripheral parts of the parenchymal nodules.

Although in theory the process may involve a single liver cell, in practice several necrotic cells need to be present before the process can be recognized with the light microscope. As is the case with focal necrosis, remnants of necrotic liver cells are not always to be found, and the necrosis is only evident because of defects of the liver cell plate structure and the presence of focal inflammation. The inflammatory infiltrate is mainly composed of lymphocytes and plasma cells, but in most cases a few neutrophils and histiocytes are also present[58, 89, 278].

The extent of piecemeal necrosis usually varies not only from portal tract to portal tract but also in different parts of a single portal tract[89, 280]. The same holds true for cirrhotic nodules. In the early stages there is no fibrosis in relation to piecemeal necrosis[265]. Later, new connective tissue is often found, especially when the necrosis is extensive[58, 164].

Morphological diagnosis: The recognition of piecemeal necrosis is as a rule easy even at lower magnifications in H & E-stained sections. It is essential to demonstrate either the necrotic liver cells or the defects of the liver cell plates, as well as infiltration by lymphocytes and plasma cells. The collapse of reticulin fibers in the periportal or periseptal zone is a good marker, but the diagnosis cannot be made on reticulin-stained sections only. The demonstration or exclusion of fibrosis in older lesions requires staining for collagen fibers.

Differential diagnosis: In livers with severe portal inflammation from any cause, "spill-over" of lymphocytes and plasma cells is often seen[93]. This spill-over merely represents inflammatory cell infiltration (Fig. 23), and the diagnosis of piecemeal necrosis can be made only when evidence of liver cell necrosis is found in addition.

In large bile duct obstruction there may also be necrosis of the peripheral parts of the lobules[291]. This necrosis is accompanied by large numbers of neutrophils (p. 186).

Additional morphological findings: Extensive piecemeal necrosis is most characteristically found in chronic aggressive hepatitis, in which it is a defining criterion[31, 58, 89]. In addition there is periportal fibrosis with bile duct proliferation and inflammatory cell infiltration. In the lobules there may be changes similar to those of acute viral hepatitis.

Piecemeal necrosis is also found in a substantial number of cases of acute viral hepatitis[265]. It is most often of minor degree but in a few per cent of biopsies more severe necrosis is seen. Fibrosis is, however, absent or minimal.

Piecemeal necrosis may also be found in Wilson's disease, in primary biliary cirrhosis[69] and in other forms of cirrhosis such as that following acute viral hepatitis[93] or chronic aggressive hepatitis[99]. It may sometimes be seen in later stages of alcoholic liver disease[66]. Mild piecemeal necrosis can in addition be observed in a variety of diseases such as infectious mononucleosis and chronic inflammatory bowel disease[106].

Occurrence and significance: As indicated above, piecemeal necrosis is most often found in chronic aggressive hepatitis and in acute viral hepatitis. When much piecemeal necrosis is seen in the latter, a suspicion of chronicity must be raised, since many such cases later develop chronic aggressive hepatitis and cirrhosis[101]. This is more often so in older people than in the young.

The degree of piecemeal necrosis can be used as an indicator of the histological activity of a chronic aggressive hepatitis, and this is usually in good agreement with clinical activity[89, 99]. Its significance in the other diseases mentioned is uncertain.

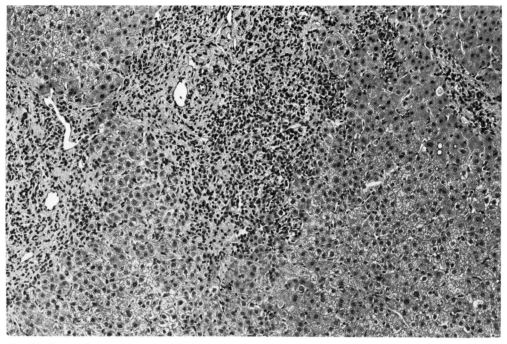

Fig. 72: Parts of two portal tracts (left side and middle) and adjacent parenchyma. The lower and right part of the central portal tract contains a great number of piecemeal necrosis with many inflammatory cells. Chronic aggressive hepatitis (Needle biopsy, H & E x 110).

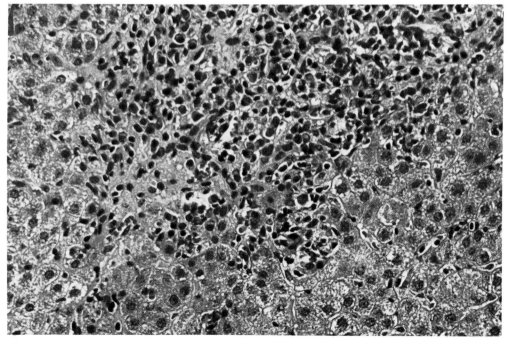

Fig. 73: Closer view of a part of the piecemeal necrosis area illustrated in Fig. 72. In addition to histiocytes, plasma cells and lymphocytes are seen. An acidophil body is present a little right of and below the center (Needle biopsy, H & E x 270).

Confluent

Morphology: Confluent necrosis is defined as necrosis of adjoining areas of liver cells[29, 143, 327a] (Fig. 74 & 75). Confluent necrosis is most often centrilobular but may also be intermediate in location or periportal[94]. In most cases this type of lesion is relatively localized, comprising only smaller parts of the lobules, but whole lobules can be affected – panlobular necrosis[15, 143, 273] (p. 88). A particular form is so-called bridging necrosis[29, 40, 77] (p. 90).

The distribution of confluent necrosis is most variable within the liver, and even in a biopsy one may sometimes find that confluent necrosis is missing in some places, while in others, the areas may be many and large, possibly panlobular.

In the early stages one usually finds remnants of necrotic cells; later the lysis is complete. The reticulin fibers are fairly well preserved[96] but since the liver cells in between the fibers disappear, condensation takes place, so-called collapse. Small areas of confluent necrosis are as a rule resorbed and replaced by complete regeneration, whereas more extensive necrosis is nearly always followed by formation of new connective tissue[176].

Confluent necrosis is always accompanied by infiltration of inflammatory cells[273]. The degree and quality of the inflammation depends to some degree on the etiology, but most often the inflammation is rather slight and dominated by histiocytes[273]. This is nearly always the case in, for instance, ischemic necrosis, necrosis arising after toxins, and also sometimes in acute hepatitis (due to both viruses and drugs). In other cases of acute hepatitis the inflammation is more pronounced and also comprises lymphocytes, plasma cells and neutrophils[94].

In the early stages confluent necrosis often has blurred borders but later, probably partly due to the inflammatory reaction, the demarcation from the adjacent liver tissue grows more distinct[273]. Well-demarcated centrilobular confluent necrosis is often conspicuous in acute hepatitis induced by halothane[262].

Morphological diagnosis: A reticulin fiber stain demonstrating areas of collapse is a good marker for the presence of confluent necrosis, but the diagnosis is made on H & E-stained sections. Serial sections are important for the evaluation of a zonal distribution, and staining for collagen fibers is necessary for the evaluation of the age of the necrosis.

Differential diagnosis: Confluent fibrosis may in its early phases look very similar to confluent necrosis, and sometimes transistional forms occur. In practice the term confluent necrosis is used when there is no fibrosis. The transitional form may be called confluent necrosis with early fibrosis, and the term confluent fibrosis is restricted to a lesion characterized by mature connective tissue and absence of liver cell remnants. Bile infarct see p. 98, and ischemic necrosis see p. 100.

Additional morphological findings: Confluent necrosis is to be found in many different diseases and may therefore be demonstrated together with a large variety of portal and parenchymal changes. Acute hepatitis is a good example[40] (p. 174). In confluent necrosis, provoked for instance by cardiac shock, sinusoidal dilatation of the adjacent parenchyma may be conspicuous and the necrosis is usually associated with hemorrhage[37, 52]. In toxic liver damage such as that due to carbon tetrachloride, the adjacent parenchyma is often fatty[187].

Occurrence and significance: The presence of confluent necrosis is a sign of severe damage of the liver parenchyma. Confluent necrosis is seen in 5–10 per cent of biopsies from patients with acute hepatitis[265] and in 20–30 per cent of chronic aggressive hepatitis[58]. Confluent necrosis may also be found after many different drugs (including halothane) and toxins (for instance carbon tetrachloride or phosphorus)[187], and in relation to shock of differing etiology and in toxemia of pregnancy[8]. Irregularly distributed confluent necrosis is sometimes seen in cirrhosis.

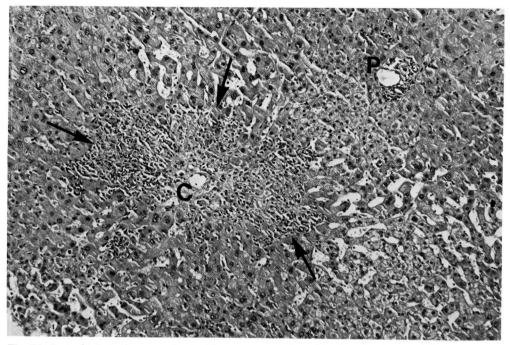

Fig. 74: Part of lobule from a patient with severe acute hepatitis. A rather large confluent necrosis around the central vein (C) is demarcated by arrows. Moderate inflammation. (Portal tract: P) (Needle biopsy, H & E x 110).

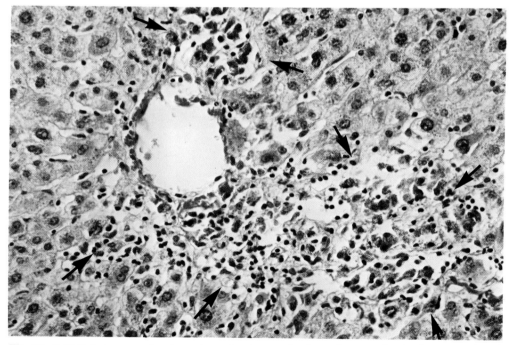

Fig. 75: Centrilobular area showing a large focal necrosis above the central vein (two arrows) and a rather small confluent necrosis below (five arrows). The inflammation is dominated by pigment-loaded macrophages. Acute hepatitis (Needle biopsy, van Gieson x 270).

Panlobular and massive

Morphology: Panlobular necrosis is confluent necrosis affecting a whole lobule. The lesion is termed multiple panlobular necrosis if many lobules are totally necrotic (Fig. 76 & 77), and massive necrosis when the whole liver is necrotic[7, 15, 94]. Panlobular and massive necrosis are thus very extensive forms of confluent necrosis; they are discussed here separately because of their special morphological and clinical implications.

The inflammatory reaction in liver tissue with panlobular or massive necrosis is usually only slight, with scattered histiocytes in the central areas and some lymphocytes and plasma cells in the periphery[274]. If the patient survives for more than about a week, an increasing number of bile-duct-like structures are seen[166]. The necrotic lobule develops into an area of collapse, often called primary collapse in contrast to the secondary collapse which follows extensive confluent necrosis in parenchymal nodules[274, 281].

In primary collapse the spatial relationship between portal tracts and central veins is preserved but all distances are reduced[274]. A sharp border is seen between the original portal tract with dense collagen fibers and the area of collapsed parenchyma.

The distribution of panlobular necrosis is most often uneven in the liver, and it is not uncommon to find, for instance, in acute viral[29, 96] or drug-induced hepatitis[262], some areas with panlobular necrosis and others both with and without confluent necrosis in the same biopsy.

All transitional stages between panlobular necrosis and panlobular fibrosis may be found.

Massive necrosis corresponds in its morphological features to panlobular necrosis, but it affects the whole or virtually the whole liver.

Morphological diagnosis: The diagnosis is to be made on sections stained with H & E and sections stained for reticulin and collagen fibers.

Prerequisites are collapse of whole lobules with diminished distances between portal tracts and central veins, complete or nearly complete lack of preserved liver cells, and absence of fibrosis.

Differential diagnosis: Once familiar with the picture one will usually find the diagnosis easy, and the lesion not readily confused with others. Staining for collagen fibers may be necessary for differentiation from panlobular fibrosis.

Additional morphological findings: In some cases all the parenchyma in a biopsy is necrotic. In others, better preserved areas exhibit features such as those found in acute hepatitis, sinusoidal dilatation and steatosis.

Occurrence and significance: Panlobular necrosis is registered in less than 1 per cent of our liver biopsy material[58, 265]. Its presence is always an expression of very severe parenchymal damage, but because of the usually uneven distribution the possibility of sampling error is very high[94, 274]. Complete necrosis of all lobules in a biopsy does thus not necessarily mean that the patient has massive necrosis[207]. Conversely, complete absence of panlobular necrosis in a biopsy does not signify that panlobular necrosis cannot be present in other areas of the liver[166].

Moreover, what has been said regarding the occurrence of confluent necrosis also holds true here.

If the patient has a true massive necrosis, hepatic coma and death will ensue[207, 273]. If the patient survives, panlobular necrosis is converted to scars, the size of which of course depends on the extent of the necrosis[176].

In addition it must be added that panlobular and/or massive necrosis may arise at any time in the course of acute[96] and chronic hepatitis[94] and of cirrhosis following hepatitis[274], though this is not common.

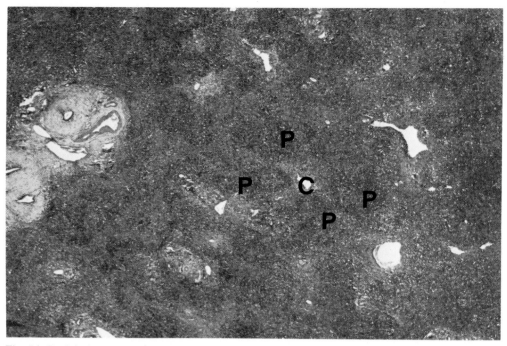

Fig. 76: Panlobular necrosis comprising many lobules. One lobule is indicated by letters (P: portal tracts, C: central vein). Note the short distances between portal tracts and/or central veins. From a patient with acute hepatitis (Surgical biopsy, H & E x 30).

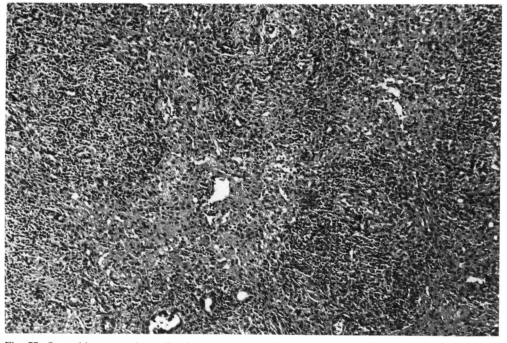

Fig. 77: Same biopsy as above. In the middle and left third a lobule with a central vein and five portal tracts is seen. The liver cells are replaced by macrophages and there is severe portal and periportal inflammation (Surgical biopsy, H & E x 110).

Bridging

Morphology: Bridging necrosis is necrosis linking central areas, portal areas or portal and central areas, and may therefore be termed central-central, portal-central (Fig. 78 & 79) or portal-portal bridging necrosis[7,31,93]. In the literature, bridging necrosis has also been called subacute hepatic necrosis[40]. The most important form is portal-central bridging necrosis[274], and if no special indication is given in the text it is this form which is meant.

Portal-central bridging necrosis has a distribution which often corresponds to Rappaport's zone 3 [7,274,301]. Bridges are as a rule unevenly distributed in the liver, often with one or two or possibly three or four in one lobule and none in the adjacent lobules. Their breadth varies from narrow necrotic zones to necrotic areas comprising the greater part of the lobule.

Multiple follow-up biopsies have indicated the probability that bridging necrosis primarily may arise as confluent necrosis in zone 3 of Rappaport's acinus[274]. In such cases the inflammation is only slight, and dominated by histiocytes. In other cases the bridging necrosis consists of piecemeal necrosis extending from the portal tracts[93,94]; gradually, over months or years, the necrosis spreads through the parenchyma to the central veins. This lesion is accompanied by many inflammatory cells, particularly lymphocytes and plasma cells.

Bridging necrosis may also, perhaps quite frequently, be comprised of a mixture of piecemeal necrosis and confluent necrosis with many lymphocytes and plasma cells periportally and rather few inflammatory cells – mainly histiocytes – around the central veins[274].

In bridging necrosis the reticulin network is usually destroyed to such a degree that complete regeneration cannot take place and bridging fibrosis develops[274].

Portal-portal bridging necrosis is a result of piecemeal necrosis and is often seen in a slender and delicate form in acute hepatitis[29,274]. Extensive portal-portal bridging necrosis is more characteristic for chronic aggressive hepatitis[31,89]. Central-central bridging necrosis is demonstrated infrequently[274].

Morphological diagnosis: A prerequisite for the diagnosis of portal-central bridging necrosis is that the necrosis actually extends from the portal tract to the central vein. Collapse of the reticulin framework can be used only as a guide, and the diagnosis must be made on H & E-stained sections and sections stained for collagen fibers. The latter are used to distinguish between bridging necrosis and bridging fibrosis. Serial sections are of great value for the evaluation of the extent of the necrosis.

Differential diagnosis: In H & E-stained sections bridging fibrosis may – particularly in the early stages – look very similar to bridging necrosis, and there are of course biopsies which show transitional forms. Corresponding to the terms used one can distinguish three stages: bridging necrosis, bridging necrosis with early fibrosis and bridging fibrosis.

Additional morphological findings: Bridging necrosis is most common in chronic aggressive hepatitis[58] and in severe forms of acute hepatitis[101,265] and, consequently, one may find the other changes of these diseases (chapter III).

Bridging necrosis has also – although only exceptionally – been recorded in cardiac insufficiency[274,360].

Occurrence and significance: In chronic aggressive hepatitis bridging necrosis has been demonstrated in more than half of the cases by use of serial biopsies[58]. The splitting up of the lobules and the subsequent development of bridging fibrosis leads to cirrhosis[99].

In consecutive series of biopsies from patients with acute hepatitis bridging necrosis is found in only a very small percentage[101]. In these cases also bridging necrosis probably plays an important role in the development of cirrhosis.

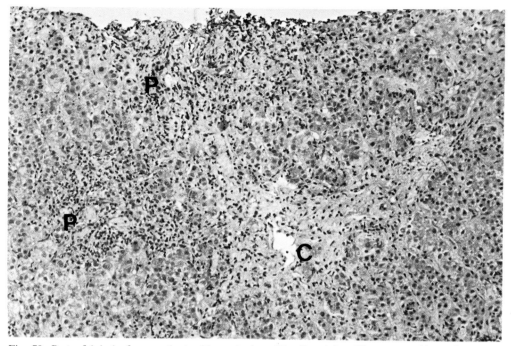

Fig. 78: Part of lobule from patient with acute hepatitis. Broad bandlike areas without liver cells connecting central vein (C) with portal tracts (P) are seen (bridging necrosis). There is moderate portal and periportal inflammation (Needle biopsy, H & E x 110).

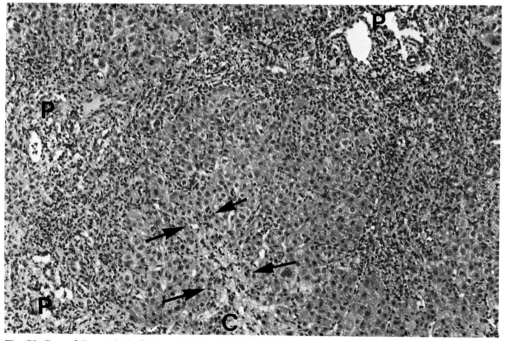

Fig. 79: Part of liver lobule from a patient with acute hepatitis with suspicion of chronicity. A narrow bridging necrosis is indicated by arrows. Many areas of piecemeal necrosis are seen. C: central vein area, P: portal tract (Needle biopsy, H & E x 110).

Alcoholic hepatitis

Morphology: In this atlas the term alcoholic hepatitis is used as a morphological diagnosis based on liver cells with Mallory bodies associated with necrosis of the same cells and with cellular and pericellular infiltration by neutrophils[56, 68, 203, 343] (Fig. 80 & 81). The necrosis is indicated by blurred cell membranes and karyopyknosis, karyolysis and karyorrhexis.

Alcoholic hepatitis may be found in a single cell with a Mallory body, in a single cell situated in a group of cells with Mallory bodies or in some or all the cells in a group[56]. Using serial sections it can be demonstrated that the neutrophils in the parenchyma are in most cases in close relation to liver cells containing Mallory bodies[56, 61].

In liver tissue from chronic alcoholics with preserved lobular architecture, the alcoholic hepatitis is usually seen in the centrilobular zone, whereas the lesions in cirrhosis are mainly localized in the periphery of the parenchymal nodules[56].

In cases with longstanding cholestasis, both Mallory bodies and alcoholic hepatitis are nearly always to be found in the peripheral parts of the lobules (periportally)[142].

Morphological diagnosis: Alcoholic hepatitis is best recognized in H & E-stained sections. When the changes are typical and extensive the diagnosis can be made even at low magnification, but otherwise it is necessary to perform a systematic evaluation of the biopsy at high magnification. The demonstration of neutrophils in the parenchyma or of liver cells with Mallory bodies always raises a suspicion of alcoholic hepatitis and serial sectioning is recommended[56]. Sections stained for collagen fibers are necessary for an accurate estimation of possible fibrosis.

Differential diagnosis: The picture of alcoholic hepatitis as defined here does not in practice give differential diagnostic difficulties, particularly when serial sections are available. The serial sections allow an assessment of the spatial relationship between neutrophils and liver cells with Mallory bodies.

Additional morphological findings: Alcoholic hepatitis is most commonly found in biopsies from chronic alcoholics, and the liver is nearly always steatotic and often cirrhotic[56, 61, 286]. When the lobular architecture is preserved, localized fibrosis is very frequent[56]. Both the fibrosis and the steatosis may be slight. The fibrosis is most often seen as pericellular fibrosis (p. 156), but central hyaline sclerosis is not rare[113] (p. 160).

Mallory bodies may also be found in some patients with longstanding cholestasis[142], and changes resembling those of alcoholic hepatitis may therefore sometimes be demonstrated in primary and secondary biliary cirrhosis and their precirrhotic stages. In addition, lesions such as those of alcoholic hepatitis have been described in liver biopsies from patients with Wilson's disease[142], and a very severe form may be present in Indian childhood cirrhosis[297, 349]. Finally, it should be mentioned that "alcoholic hepatitis" has also been demonstrated in some biopsies from patients after an intestinal by-pass operation for obesity[263].

Occurrence and significance: Alcoholic hepatitis is present in a very substantial part of most series of alcoholic cirrhosis[60, 66], and it is generally accepted that alcoholic hepatitis is the most important factor in the development of cirrhosis in alcoholics[64].

The significance of alcoholic hepatitis in the other conditions mentioned above is less clear[142].

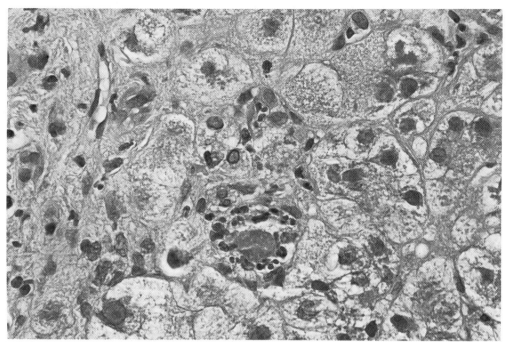

Fig. 80: Alcoholic hepatitis. In the lower part of the middle third of the picture a clumpformed Mallory body is seen. It is surrounded by a light zone with debris and with neutrophils and macrophages. From an alcoholic with cirrhosis (Needle biopsy, H & E x 400).

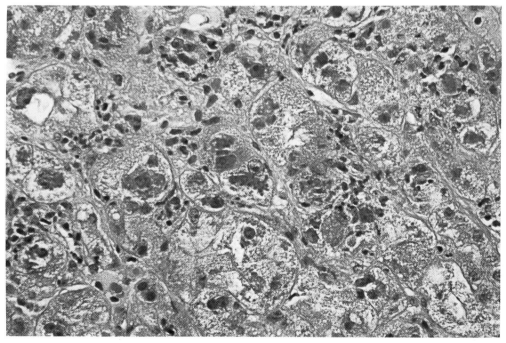

Fig. 81: Slightly lower magnification of another area of the same biopsy as above. Many Mallory bodies with varying size and shape are seen within necrotic or non-necrotic liver cells (Needle biopsy, H & E x 270).

Lipogranulomas

Morphology: Lipogranulomas are granulomatous structures comprising one or more extracellular lipid droplets surrounded by lymphocytes and histiocytes and often by many eosinophils[57, 264] (Fig. 82). In the early stages of the development of the granulomas the amount of cytoplasm of the histiocytes is sparse, but later the cells have the appearance of lipophages or epithelioid cells, and giant cells may be formed. Collagen fibers are few or absent.

Lipogranulomas occur focally, singly, or in small groups and are encountered in all parts of the lobules where the liver cells contain fat. The number of lipogranulomas varies from one or very few per biopsy to several per lobule. If many lipogranulomas are present they are usually evenly distributed throughout the biopsy, though focal accumulations are sometimes seen.

Multinodular structures built up of confluent small lipogranulomas are observed in a minority of cases [57] (Fig. 83). These structures differ from the small ones not only in size but also because they frequently lie in close relation to the central vein and because there nearly always are collagen fibers in and between the individual nodules.

Morphological diagnosis: Lipogranulomas are easily recognized even at low magnification in H & E-stained sections. The centrally located vacuole, most often with blurred margins, and the histiocytic reaction are characteristic. Staining for collagen fibers is necessary to evaluate the amount of connective tissue. Stainings for fat are not of any value in paraffin embedded material.

Differential diagnosis: Lipogranulomas have in general a typical appearance but can in some cases, when the picture is dominated by epithelioid cell-like lipophages, be nearly impossible to distinguish from actual epithelioid cell granulomas[170] (p. 42). The most reliable way to separate the lipogranulomas from the latter is by the use of serial sections to demonstrate fat vacuoles. Another important criterion is the the invariably intralobular location of lipogranulomas[57, 170].

Additional morphological findings: When lipogranulomas are present in a biopsy the parenchyma is virtually always steatotic[57]. In the very rare cases where lipogranulomas are found without steatosis, the reason, in our experience, is that when the effect of the provoking etiological agent ceases the steatosis soon diminishes, whereas it takes a longer time to resolve the lipogranulomas.

Since alcohol is one of the most common causes of steatosis, lipogranulomas are *ipso facto* often associated with alcoholic hepatitis and cirrhosis[65, 66].

Occurrence and significance: Lipogranulomas are, as stated above, commonly found and undoubtedly arise from rupture of one or more steatotic liver cells. They may be recognized in all patients with steatosis but are most frequently observed in alcoholics[57, 66].

In our material we have estimated that in biopsies with "pure steatosis" (i.e. without cirrhosis, cholestasis, Mallory bodies, etc.) lipogranulomas are to be found in one half to one third[57]. The biopsies with lipogranulomas show greater histological activity (focal necrosis, acidophil bodies and mesenchymal reaction) than the biopsies without[57].

Whereas fibrosis is minimal or absent in relation to small lipogranulomas, the amount of collagen fibers in and around large lipogranulomas is sometimes considerable, and it is probable that these multinodular structures in some cases play a significant role in the development of cirrhosis[57].

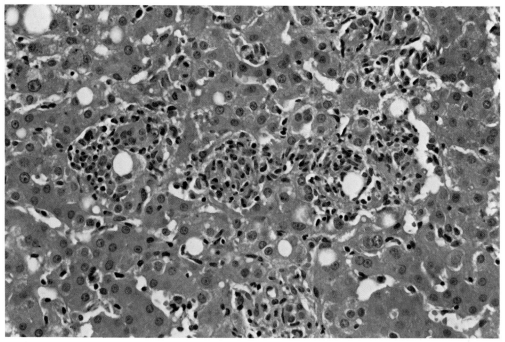

Fig. 82: Small lipogranulomas with many eosinophils. Of the three granulomas seen in the equatorial zone of the picture, two show a central vacuole, the third (middle) is without. Serial sections disclosed a vacuole in the latter (Needle biopsy, H & E x 270).

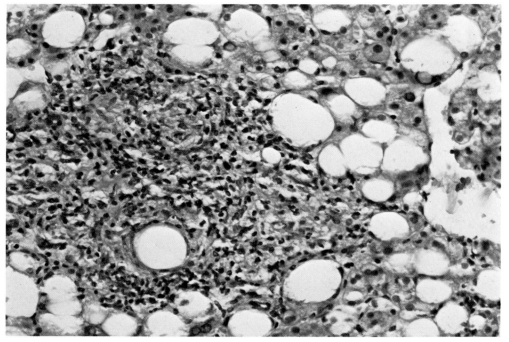

Fig. 83: Large lipogranuloma with fibrosis and inflammatory cells. The lesion has a nodular structure and is not sharply delimited. Part of a central vein is seen in the right part of the picture (Needle biopsy, H & E x 270).

Focal necrosis with neutrophils

Morphology: Focal liver cell necrosis with neutrophils is seen as defects of liver cells plates just as focal liver cell necrosis with Kupffer cell proliferation. The inflammatory reaction is, however, dominated by neutrophils[70, 194]. The focal defects are usually small and comprise only a few liver cells. In the earliest stages remnants of liver cell nuclei and cytoplasm may be demonstrable but complete lysis quickly develops. In addition to neutrophils a few lymphocytes and histiocytes may be present.

Focal liver cell necrosis with neutrophils most often is found in liver biopsies performed during the late stages of an operation in the upper abdomen[70, 194] (Fig. 84 & 85). This type is here termed surgical necrosis and is to be found in both wedge and needle biopsies. Since in many centers it is more common to perform wedge biopsies than needle biopsies during operation, the lesion is more commonly found in the former.

Surgical necrosis is widely distributed throughout the liver. The earliest changes are found in the centrilobular zone, often adjacent to the central vein, and in the subcapsular areas.

Focal liver cell necrosis with neutrophils may in addition be found in other conditions such as obstruction of large bile ducts[67, 291, 293]and, more rarely, sepsis and pyemia[296]. In obstruction of the large bile ducts the changes mainly occur in or close to the limiting plate; they are nearly always small but when there are many, destruction of the limiting plate may take place[67, 291, 293].

In septicemic and pyemic conditions the lesions are more irregularly distributed in the parenchyma; usually some are large and comprise many liver cells[296] (abscess formation).

(Focal liver cell necrosis with Mallory bodies and neutrophils: see alcoholic hepatitis, p. 92).

Morphological diagnosis: The diagnosis of focal liver cell necrosis with neutrophils is in general relatively easy in sections stained with H & E, in particular when changes are severe. A prerequisite for the diagnosis is that there are, in addition to neutrophils, defects of the liver cell plates.

Differential diagnosis: It is always easy to differentiate between focal liver cell necrosis with neutrophils and focal necrosis with Kupffer cell proliferation. On the other hand the lesion in question may give problems in differentiation from alcoholic hepatitis[61]. The use of multiple sections is necessary to exclude the presence of Mallory bodies.

Additional morphological findings: Surgical necrosis arises in the late stages of an operation, and it may therefore be found in otherwise normal liver tissue and in livers with all types of changes[70]. The same holds true for the necrosis developing in septicemic and pyemic conditions[296]. (Large duct obstruction, see p. 186).

Occurrence and significance: Surgical necrosis is found in one third to one half of all biopsies performed in the late stages of upper abdominal operations[70]. The lesions probably arise as a result of anoxia and are probably of no clinical significance[70, 194, 365]. Severe surgical necrosis with many and large lesions may, however, disturb the morphological picture and provoke difficulties in the interpretation of a possible primary liver disease. It is recommended, that the liver biopsy be performed early during the operation.

Periportal focal liver cell necrosis with neutrophils in combination with portal changes such as marginal bile duct proliferation, edema and infiltration by neutrophils and centrilobular cholestasis speaks in favor of large duct obstruction[67, 291].

Irregularly distributed focal necrosis together with neutrophils of varying sizes gives a strong suspicion of a septic or pyemic condition[296].

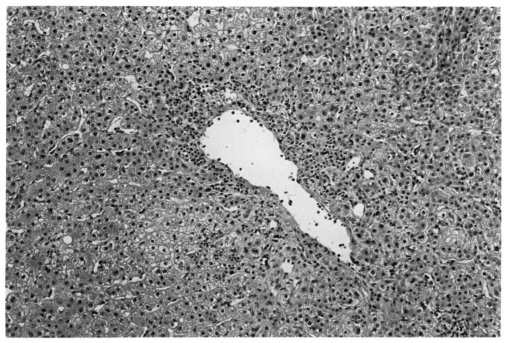

Fig. 84: "Surgical" necrosis from a biopsy taken late during an operation. Many small rounded or polygonal defects of the liver cell plates replaced by neutrophils are seen, mainly in the neighborhood of the sublobular vein (Surgical biopsy, H & E x 110).

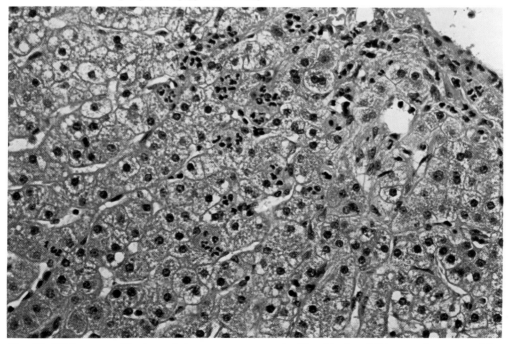

Fig. 85: Higher magnification of the same areas as in Fig. 84. In addition to the neutrophils, one can see cellular debris in some of the defects of the liver cell plates (Surgical biopsy, H & E x 270).

Bile infarct

Morphology: A bile infarct is a necrosis of smaller or larger areas of adjoining liver cells in association with – probably bile-induced – cytoplasmic changes (Fig. 86 & 87). The smaller infarcts, comprising only a few cells, may be found in all forms of severe cholestasis and in all parts of the lobule, whereas the larger ones are periportal and most often seen in connection with obstruction of the larger bile ducts.

Initially, small groups of swollen liver cells with a strongly vacuolated cytoplasm giving a characteristic netlike pattern are seen. The change is called feathery or xanthomatous degeneration[138, 282] (p. 106). The cytoplasm of these cells may gradually acquire a green color as a result of intracellular bile accumulation[318]. Later the cellular boundaries and the nuclei fade away, sometimes after a period of karyopyknosis. The necrosis calls forth only slight inflammatory reaction[273]. The reticulin network is intact for a relatively long time but subsequently progressive fragmentation takes place. Fibrin deposits may be conspicuous.

As a rule the bile disappears from the area, and a common picture is that of a light area with so-called ghost cells[327d].

Morphological diagnosis: A young bile infarct comprising areas of necrotic, bile impregnated liver cells is easily recognized even at small magnification. The older infarcts are best recognized by the ghost cells.

Differential diagnosis: The true bile infarct must be distinguished from xanthomatous degeneration of the liver cells. This lesion forms part of the earliest changes in the development of the bile infarct but the degeneration is not always followed by necrosis[282, 327d].

The appearance of both the early bile impregnated infarct and the late infarct dominated by ghost cells is as a rule so characteristic that is should not be confused with any other lesion. A bile lake arises after rupture of dilated portal bile ducts and consequently occurs in the portal tracts[327e]. The changes may overlap the parenchyma but the most pronounced components, the bile deposits, the inflammation and the frequently found granulomatous reaction are mainly located in the portal tracts.

Additional morphological findings: Bile infarcts occur in patients with severe cholestasis and most often following large duct obstruction[327e] (p. 186). Whereas we most often found large infarcts in relation to the latter, small bile infarcts may in addition be observed in intrahepatic cholestasis[293]. Thus we have seen small bile infarcts in a few cases of acute hepatitis due to virus or drugs (p. 174). Bile infarcts have also, though exceptionally, been demonstrated in cirrhosis, especially primary biliary cirrhosis.

Occurrence and significance: Bile infarcts are only registered in a very small proportion of liver biopsies, and they have consequently only limited value in routine diagnostic work. Large bile infarcts give a strong suspicion of large duct obstruction[327e], whereas small infarcts may be seen in severe cholestasis from any cause[293].

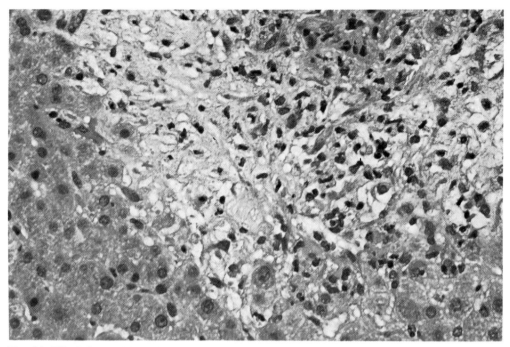

Fig. 86: Bile infarct without bile. Normal appearing liver cells are seen in the left side and the lower part of the picture. In between the xanthomatous cells a few inflammatory cells are found. Large duct obstruction (Needle biopsy, H & E x 270).

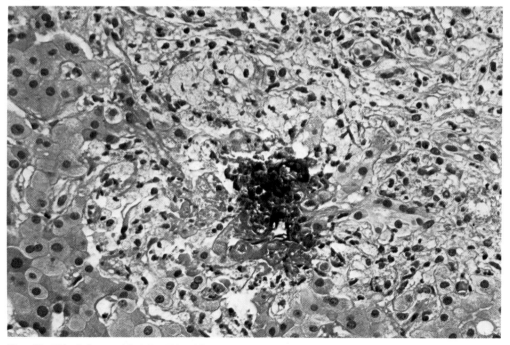

Fig. 87: Bile infarct with bile. The bile is dark and the color ranges from orange to green and black. Left of the bile precipitate eosinophil cellular debris and fibrin are present. Large duct obstruction (Surgical biopsy, H & E x 270).

Ischemic

Morphology: Ischemic liver cell necrosis is a type of coagulative necrosis which characteristically comprises swollen liver cells with partly preserved contours but with eosinophilic, homogeneous cytoplasm and varying degrees of karyopyknosis, karyorrhexis and karyolysis[51, 273] (Fig. 88 & 89).

This type of necrosis is as a rule sharply demarcated but may have all sizes and shapes. When present in cirrhosis the lesion can affect small groups of cells, whole nodules or groups of nodules[51]. In livers with normal architecture the delineation is irregular and seems to be without special relation to be the lobules or acini[327h].

In the outer zones of the ischemic necrosis and sometimes also in the visible remnants of the sinusoids, infiltration by histiocytes and in particular neutrophils is present. The inflammation is characteristically slight in this type of necrosis and without significant hemorrhage[273].

The contour of the cells only become blurred slowly[273]. Fibrosis may develop.

Morphology diagnosis: The histologic picture is very characteristic and the lesion is easily diagnosed in H & E-stained sections, usually even at low magnifications.

Differential diagnosis: An ischemic necrosis of the liver cells may in the later stages look somewhat similar to confluent necrosis. In the former, however, contours of the liver cells are better preserved and there is usually less inflammation[273]. Furthermore the neutrophils are the predominant cells. In livers with preserved architectures, confluent necrosis usually has zonal distribution[273] and this is not the case with ischemic necrosis[327h]. In cirrhotic livers the size and shape of the two types of necrosis may be identical.

Additional morphological findings: Ischemic necrosis is most commonly found in cirrhosis[51] and in liver cell tumors, both adenoma and carcinoma[48]. It may arise in all types of cirrhosis. It is rare to find thrombosis.

Occurrence and significance: Ischemic necrosis only rarely occurs in biopsies. When found in cirrhosis it often, though not always, follows gastro-intestinal bleeding[273].

In liver cell adenomas smaller or larger areas of coagulative necrosis are often present[48]. It is probable that the necrosis provokes the intra-abdominal hemorrhage not uncommon in these patients.

The occurrence of ischemic necrosis in a biopsy from a non-cirrhotic liver should always raise suspicion of a liver cell tumor and, if necessary, serial sections should be examined.

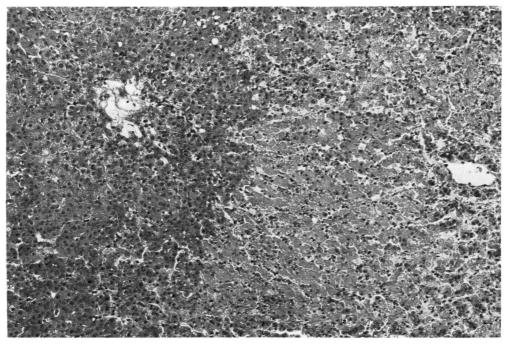

Fig. 88: Coagulative necrosis with swollen, granular liver cells, without cellular details. The liver cell plates can still be recognized. There is only slight inflammation. In the left half of the picture the liver cells show preserved details (Surgical biopsy, H & E x 110).

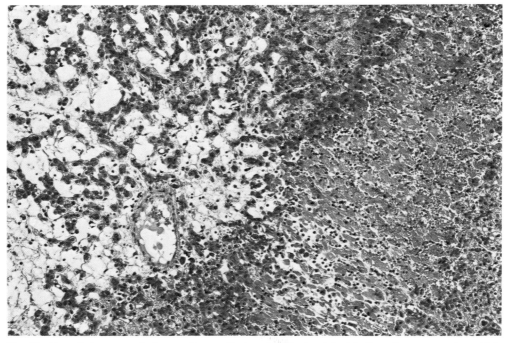

Fig. 89: Coagulative necrosis from a liver cell adenoma. In the left side there is a severe sinusoidal dilatation in relation to which the liver cell plates are atrophic. The liver cells in the atrophic plates are without necrosis (Surgical biopsy, H & E x 110).

Abnormal

Morphology: The liver cell nuclei may deviate from normal in different ways. The number of nuclei in a single cell may be increased, the nuclear size may vary more than normal, and the nuclear structure may be altered.

In normal liver tissue only few cells with two or more nuclei are observed[72] but in a series of parenchymal liver diseases – in particular acute hepatitis[298] – the number of liver cells with two or more nuclei is enhanced. In the special giant cell hepatitis seen in children greatly enlarged liver cells with up to 10 or more nuclei are common[155, 320] (Fig. 90).

Most of the liver cells in normal liver tissue are diploid but both tetraploid and octaploid cells are to be found[123]. An increased number of liver cells with enlarged nuclei are very frequent in acute hepatitis[29, 166, 265, 298]. The nucleoli are in addition often conspicuous.

So-called nuclear vacuoles are in fact invaginations of the nuclear membrane since ultrastructural investigations have shown that they contain cytoplasmic components and serial sections have demonstrated connections with the cytoplasm[197]. In the light microscope they are seen as intranuclear vacuoles which are either optically empty or contain granular material.

So-called glycogen nuclei are seen in H & E-stained sections as optically empty nuclei with condensation of chromatin elements on the inner side of the nuclear membrane[327k]. Electron microscopically large amounts of glycogen are visible and light microscopically PAS staining is positive (Fig. 91).

So-called "sanded nuclei" are found as isolated or small groups of weakly stained, slightly granular nuclei (Fig. 90). Ultrastruturally closely set core particles are demonstrated[33].

Inclusion bodies of cytomegal-virus are sometimes present in both liver cells and bile duct epithelium[154]. They appear basophilic in H & E-stained sections and are typically surrounded by a light "halo" (Fig. 91).

Morphological diagnosis: Nuclear changes are best determined on H & E-stained sections. The recognition of small changes in nuclear size may be difficult because of normal variation, and demands some experience. The number of nuclei per cell also shows some variation in normal livers but the occurrence of liver cells with three nuclei or more, or more than 3–4 liver cells with two nuclei per lobule, may be regarded as pathological[123].

Glycogen vacuoles are not always positive after PAS staining when the biopsy is fixed in aqueous formalin. Inclusion bodies are positive in DNA-stained sections. Sanded nuclei are easily overlooked in H & E-stained sections.

Differential diagnosis: Immunological or ultrastructural demonstration of $HB_C Ag$ is necessary for the correct diagnosis of sanded nuclei.

Additional morphological findings: An increased number of liver cells with more and enlarged nuclei is in particular seen in the fully developed stage of acute hepatitis[166, 265, 289] but is also found in active periods of chronic aggressive hepatitis[58] and cirrhosis[63]. Vacuoles with cytoplasmic components are often to be demonstrated in the same conditions. Many glycogen nuclei may be seen in otherwise normal liver tissue[327k] as well as in a large number of different pathological conditions such as steatosis, non-specific reactive hepatitis and cirrhosis and diabetes mellitus[351]. Sanded nuclei may be seen in chronic hepatitis and non-specific reactive hepatitis[33].

Occurrence and significance: Multinucleated liver cells, variation in nuclear size and mitoses are expressions of regenerative processes and are, as indicated above, usually found in diseases with extensive liver cell necrosis. Multinucleated cells and variation in size of the nuclei are mainly characteristic for hepatitis[29, 265], whereas many mitoses are particularly characteristic for mononucleosis.

Nuclear vacuoles[197] and glycogen nuclei[354] are expressions of degeneration and can be seen in all diseases with liver damage. Both findings are non-specific. Inclusion bodies of cytomegalovirus type are found in some cases of cytomegalic inclusion disease[154], and sanded nuclei indicate extensive HB_c formation.

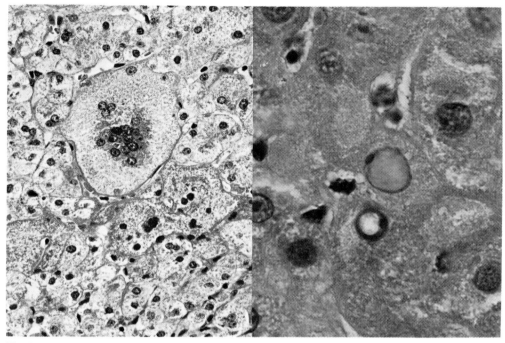

Fig. 90: Left. Multinucleated giant liver cell from a child with giant cell hepatitis (Needle biopsy, H & E x 110). Right. Sanded nucleus from a patient with chronic persistent hepatitis B (Needle biopsy, H & E x 110).

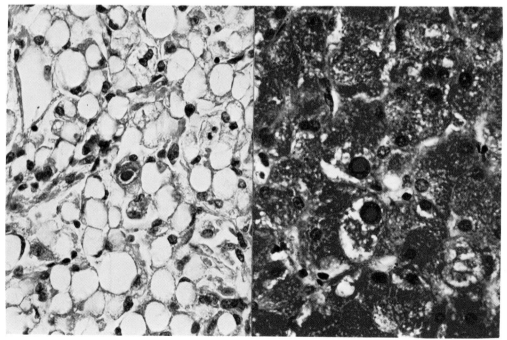

Fig. 91: Left. Intranuclear inclusion body from an infant with cytomegalic inclusion disease (Autopsy, H & E x 110). Right. Glycogen nuclei (Needle biopsy, PAS x 270).

Ballooning

Morphology: The affected cell is swollen, up to several times its normal size[219]. The cytoplasm appears granular but often there are empty looking areas in the peripheral part of the cell. The granules are minute and faintly eosinophilic, and are usually most closely packed around the nucleus[403] (Fig. 92). The cytoplasm may also contain a few granules of bile pigment. The cell membrane is often distinct but may be blurred by focal lysis, permitting the contents of two liver cells to merge[87]. The nucleus is most frequently enlarged with a loose structure. Cells with more than one nucleus are common in the more severe forms of ballooning (Fig. 93), and in rare cases the ballooned hepatocyte may be in mitosis.

Ballooning of the liver cells may be slight or severe and of varying extent. It is very often mainly centrilobular but may involve whole lobules, and in cirrhosis there are no special locations. Ballooning is commonly found in rosettes[267] (p. 72).

All transitional stages between ballooning and lytic necrosis of the liver cells may be demonstrated[273, 316]. Nuclear changes such as karyolysis and pyknosis and destruction of the cell membrane are indicative of necrosis. In addition the necrotic cell is surrounded by lymphocytes and histiocytes (p. 82). It is very probable that the slighter degrees of ballooning are reversible. Ballooning is by itself without doubt a degeneration, i.e. a retrograde change, and slight ballooning corresponds to so-called cloudy swelling[403] (syn. parenchymatous degeneration) and severe ballooning to hydropic degeneration[316].

Morphological diagnosis: Moderate and severe ballooning can in most cases be identified at low magnifications in H & E-stained sections, but slight changes may be difficult to recognize and greater magnification is necessary.

Differential diagnosis: Artefacts provoked by insufficient fixation are most often seen in the marginal zone of the biopsy and should cause no differential diagnostic problems.

Xanthomatous degeneration or feathery degeneration[282] (p. 106) seen in connection with cholestasis usually affects small groups of cells surrounded by cells which appear normal. In xanthomatous degeneration the cells are swollen but with a small pyknotic nucleus and a finely reticulated cytoplasm. In addition xanthomatous degeneration most often occurs in the peripheral parts of the lobule.

Liver cells containing Mallory bodies are usually swollen with a light, empty looking cytoplasm without the characteristic granules of ballooning[56].

Additional morphological findings: Ballooning degeneration indicates that substantial liver damage is taking place, and it is most often found in acute hepatitis accompanied by focal necrosis, acidophil bodies, and proliferation of Kupffer cells[265, 289]. Cirrhosis and chronic hepatitis with histological signs of activity also show ballooning, often to a severe degree[58].

Occurrence and significance: Slight degrees of ballooning are very commonly found in liver biopsies and are of no definite diagnostic significance. Severe, mainly centrilobular ballooning does, however, give rise to a strong suspicion of acute hepatitis and this change is a condition sine qua non for the diagnosis[29, 265] (p. 172). Severe, usually more irregularly distributed ballooning may, however, also be seen in a variety of other conditions, for instance in alcoholics[56].

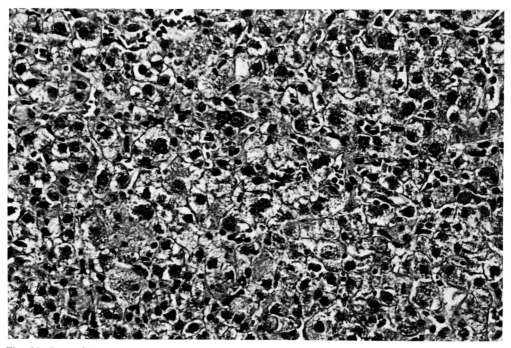

Fig. 92: Part of liver lobule from a patient with acute hepatitis. There is a slight ballooning of many liver cells, and in some places a slight focal Kupffer cell proliferation is seen (Needle biopsy, H & E x 270).

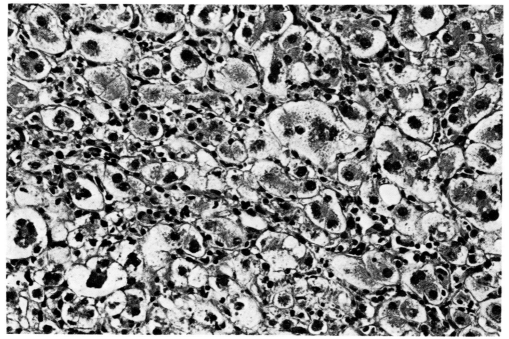

Fig. 93: Severe ballooning of most of the liver cells. In addition focal liver cell necrosis and focal Kupffer cell proliferation are seen. From a patient with acute hepatitis (Needle biopsy, H &E x 270).

Xanthomatous degeneration

Morphology: The affected cells are swollen, rounded or slightly polygonal, with a fine, conspicuous cell border. The cytoplasm is abundant, stained very pale and with a feathery or net-like pattern (Fig. 94 & 95). The fine strands contain granules of bile pigment and usually have a greenish or brownish color[282, 327d]. The nuclei appear normal or diminished in size, in the latter case often with increased staining properties.

The change may affect isolated liver cells lying among apparently normal ones, but most often smaller or larger groups of cells are involved[327d]. Xanthomatous degeneration is in most cases localized in the periportal zone. In the same area one often finds enlarged Kupffer cells, with a more or less similar appearance. Infiltration with neutrophils may be found especially when the lesion is located close to portal tracts.

When large groups of cells are changed it is common to find precipitation of bile and necrosis centrally[327d] (see bile infarct). Xanthomatous degeneration is probably induced by intracellular cholestasis, and all transitional forms to necrosis may be demonstrated[282].

Morphological diagnosis: Xanthomatous degeneration is easily identiffied in H & E-stained sections. The extent of the lesion can only be determined with some degree of certainty with the use of serial sections. Bile granules are best recognized in sections stained for iron or with van Gieson.

Differential diagnosis: Ballooning degeneration[25, 316] (p. 104) may cause differential diagnostic problems, but in these cases the enlarged cells contain a fine granular cytoplasm and enlarged nuclei and in additon the surrounding parenchyma most often shows signs of acute hepatitis (p. 172).

Additional morphological findings: Xanthomatous degeneration is seen in connection with cholestasis most often in cases with complete or nearly complete large-duct obstruction of long duration[282, 327d]. In these cases portal changes with edema, neutrophils and marginal bile duct proliferation are marked[67, 291] (p. 186). For bile infarcts, see p. 98.

Xanthomatous degeneration may also be found occasionally in parenchymal liver diseases such as pure cholestasis and acute hepatitis with pronounced cholestasis[293].

Occurrence and significance: Xanthomatous degeneration is an expression of severe and long standing cholestasis[327d]. It is, especially in more pronounced forms, mainly associated with large duct obstruction[327d]. It is, however, not uncommon in the late stages of primary biliary cirrhosis[279, 325].

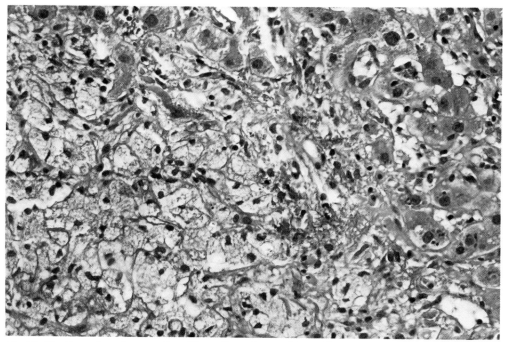

Fig. 94: Xanthomatous degeneration. The cells are large with small dark nuclei and rich in cytoplasm. The latter has a loose architecture. The cell borders are conspicuous (Needle biopsy, H & E x 270).

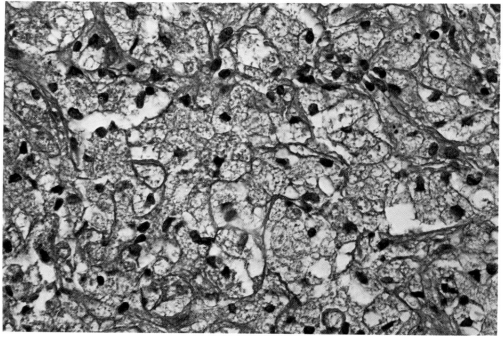

Fig. 95: Higher magnification of the same biopsy as Fig. 94. The feathery or netlike pattern of the cytoplasm is pronounced. From a patient with large duct obstruction (Needle biopsy, H & E x 400).

Steatosis

Morphology: Steatosis or fatty change is defined as light microscopically visible fat in the liver. Definitive identification of the material requires one of the lysochromes, for instance, oil red O or Sudan black B on frozen sections[206]. In practice the diagnosis of steatosis is, however, made by the finding of empty, round vacuoles in the cytoplasm of liver cells in routinely stained paraffin sections.

The size of the vacuoles varies from scarcely visible to many microns, the larger vacuoles distending the cell and displacing the nucleus to one side. The fat vacuoles are usually larger than 5–6 µm, although there is always some variation. In a minority of biopsies multiple fine vacuoles, giving the liver cells a foamy appearance, dominate the picture[195].

The degree of steatosis varies from biopsy to biopsy. In the slightest degree only a few vacuoles are found in the whole biopsy, whereas in the most severe cases every liver cell may be affected. For practical purposes it is valuable to grade the steatosis as slight, moderate or severe[158].

The localization of the fatty change may also vary (Fig. 96 & 97). In most cases there is a diffuse distribution or a centrilobular preponderance. Mainly periportal steatosis is rare, and mainly intermediate steatosis extremely rare.

Fat droplets from neighboring cells may coalesce to a large fatty cyst which lies extracellularly and produces an inflammatory reaction[57] (lipogranulomas, p. 94).

The described morphological changes are preceded by fat accumulation which can only be demonstrated chemically, and not until there is an about three- to five-fold increase in the hepatic triglyceride does fat become morphologically visible[368].

Morphological diagnosis: The diagnosis can be made on sections stained with H & E. The registration of the localization and extent of steatosis is best done at low magnifications, whereas the details and possible inflammatory reaction are best seen at higher magnifications.

Sections stained for collagen fibers are especially important for the evaluation of pericellular and focal fibrosis.

Differential diagnosis: The diagnosis is as a rule easy and the change should not be confused with other lesions.

Additional morphological findings: Steatosis may give rise to the formation of lipogranulomas[57] but provokes no other morphological changes *per se*. The additional morphological findings are to be interpreted as "parallel" effects arising at the same time[56]. Since ethanol is one of the most common causes of steatosis, the lesion is often associated with alcoholic hepatitis and cirrhosis[62]. Vacuolated nuclei seem to be more frequent in fatty change following diabetes mellitus than in other forms[351].

Occurrence and significance: Fatty change occurs in more than three fourths of alcoholics admitted to hospital[66]. As stated above, the steatosis is reversible. It is, however, often associated with other changes such as alcoholic hepatitis. When severe, the latter is often followed by formation of bridging fibrosis and eventual development of cirrhosis[63].

Fatty change in diabetics is similar to that in the alcoholic[25]. A lack of Mallory bodies and alcoholic hepatitis and the presence of vacuolated nuclei are etiologic indicators. A moderate to severe steatosis is often present in patients with marked obesity[306]. Corticoid therapy[327g] and malnutrition[79] (e.g. Kwashiorkor) may produce fatty change.

A predominantly periportal steatosis occurs in a few alcoholics[66], in some cases of active tuberculosis[172], and in alpha-l-antitrypsin deficiency[132].

The finely vacuolated type of steatosis is characteristic of the rare cases of fatty liver of pregnancy[195], Reye's syndrome[46, 249], Wilson's disease[361], and of tetracycline-induced fatty liver[261]. Fine fat droplets may also be found in glycogenosis[218].

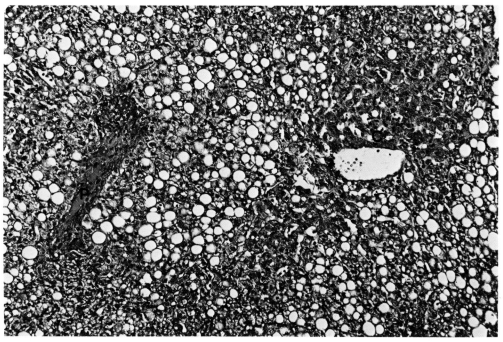

Fig. 96: Part of lobule showing moderate to severe steatosis. There is a slight periportal overweight of the steatosis (portal tract: left, central vein: right) (Needle biopsy, H & E x 110).

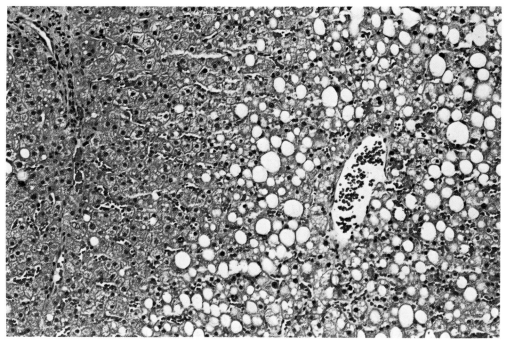

Fig. 97: Part of lobule showing moderate steatosis. There is a pronounced centrilobular overweight of the steatosis (portal tract: upper left, central vein: right) (Needle biopsy, H & E x 110).

Mallory bodies

Morphology: Alcoholic hyalin, Mallory's hyalin, or Mallory bodies appear light microscopically as eosinophilic, homogeneous masses forming irregular structures of varying size and form[56, 221] (Fig. 98 & 99). They are located in the cytoplasm of the liver cells, and the larger bodies nearly fill the cell and may have a weakly stained center surrounded by a strongly eosinophilic zone[211].

The degree of eosinophilia of Mallory bodies varies considerably from biopsy to biopsy, and to a smaller extent in the same biopsy[211]. Some are clumped, often they are worm-like, with a twisted structure. Horseshoe-shaped forms are common, and even ringformed alcoholic hyalin may be seen. The bodies are frequently excentrically situated in the cell, and characteristically the horseshoe-shaped form surrounds the nucleus at some distance with the concavity directed toward the nucleus[56].

Liver cells with Mallory bodies are as a rule enlarged, often vacuolated, with a weakly stained cytoplasm. Around the bodies a clear zone is common. The nuclei may by hyperhromatic, and sometimes the whole cell is shrunken with a fragmented or indistinct nucleus, and completely filled with hyaline masses. Liver cells with Mallory bodies occur focally, singly, or in small groups and appear in all areas of the lobule or parenchymal nodules. Most often they are seen in relation to the central veins in liver tissue with preserved architecture, and at the margins of cirrhotic nodules. The number of cells with alcoholic hyalin varies from one per biopsy to several per high power field[56].

Morphological diagnosis: The recognition of Mallory bodies is best made in H & E-stained sections and special staining techniques are unnecessary for their demonstration[56]. When the changes are extensive they can already be seen at low magnification but in all other cases a systematic search at high magnification is necessary.

Differential diagnosis: Mallory bodies generally have a typical appearance and only three other lesions need to be considered. These are acidophil bodies (p. 80), diastase-resistant PAS-positive globules (p. 114), and so-called hyaline bodies (p. 126).

Acidophil bodies are transformed whole liver cells expelled from the plates[191]. They are of the size of or smaller than liver cells, with or without nuclear remnants.

Diastase-resistant PAS-positive globules are eosinophilic, circular or oval, and are found in the cytoplasm of the liver cells (p. 204).

The hyaline bodies are sharply delineated, rounded, intracytoplasmic, eosinophillic structures[36]. They are most often 1 to 4 µm across, with a narrow translucent halo. PAS-staining is negative.

Additional morphological findings: Mallory bodies may be seen in liver tissue without alcoholic hepatitis, but only rarely[61]. The liver is most often cirrhotic but the presence of Mallory bodies in liver tissue with preserved lobular architecture is by no means uncommon[66]. In the latter cases so-called central hyaline sclerosis is frequent[113] (p. 160). Focal and pericellular fibrosis are also common in biopsies with alcoholic hyalin[63]. Steatosis is a nearly constant finding but the two lesions are hardly ever found in the same cell[55].

Occurrence and significance: Mallory bodies are most often seen in biopsies from chronic alcoholics, and it is probable that a daily, longlasting consumption is of importance for their development[60].

Mallory bodies may in addition be found in biopsies from non-alcoholic patients with long-standing cholestasis[142]. In these cases the Mallory bodies are usually located periportally in the non-cirrhotic liver, in contrast to the mainly centrilobular position in alcoholism[56]. Long-standing cholestasis with development of Mallory bodies is most typically seen in primary biliary cirrhosis and large duct obstruction, in both cases in the non-cirrhotic as well as the cirrhotic stage[142].

Mallory bodies may also be found in Wilson's disease[142], Indian childhood cirrhosis[297, 349], liver cell carcinoma[111b] and in unusual cases of by-pass operation for obesity[263].

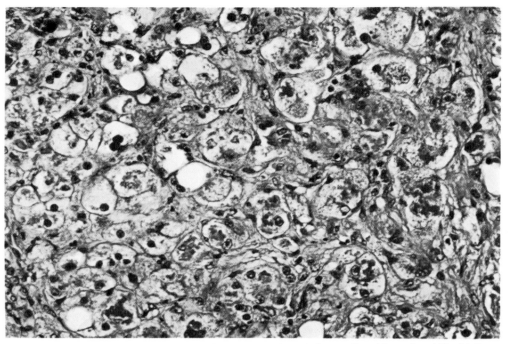

Fig. 98: Part of cirrhotic nodule comprising many enlarged liver cells with eosinophilic Mallory bodies of different sizes and shapes. No necrosis is seen. Chronic alcoholic (Needle biopsy, H & E x 270).

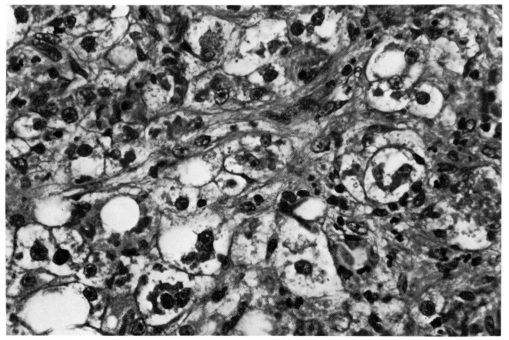

Fig. 99: Higher magnification of Mallory bodies. Two are horseshoe-shaped (lower left and middle right) while others are wormlike or quite irregular. Same biopsy as Fig. 98 (Needle biopsy, H & E x 400).

Excess glycogen

Morphology: Normal liver cells contain large but varying amounts of glycogen, which can be demonstrated both ultrastructurally and light microscopically[213]. In conditions with a pronounced increase of glycogen there is a hepatomegaly caused by an enlargement of the individual liver cells[218]. The glycogen accumulation is diffuse in the cytoplasm, and the cells are large with a palely staining cytoplasm and distinct cell borders, giving an appearance of plant cells (Fig. 100 & 101).

In most types of glycogen storage disease – so-called glycogenosis – the cells appear as described above but in the type II glycogenosis[226] the cytoplasm contains a large number of 1–2 μm vacuoles dispersed evenly throughout the cytoplasm. In glycogenosis the number of liver cells with glycogen accumulation may vary from area to area in the biopsy, but usually all cells are abnormal[226].

Hepatocellular adenoma[177] and focal nodular hyperplasia as a rule contain areas with more glycogen in the cells than is found in normal liver cells (p. 194). Glycogen is often to be found in varying and increased amounts in hepatocellular carcinoma[228] and especially in the clear cell variant the glycogen content is very high.

Cytoplasmic glycogen may also be somewhat increased in diabetics, particularly in the presence of hyperglycemia.

Morphological diagnosis: An excess of glycogen in the cytoplasm of the liver cells can be suspected on H & E-stained sections but a final diagnosis is to be made on PAS-stained sections with and without diastase digestion.

The amount of glycogen in a biopsy does not only depend on the true content but also on the fixation. The most common fixative is watery, neutralized formalin, and after a long fixation time all or nearly all glycogen may disappear from the cells.

Differential diagnosis: The normal content of glycogen in the liver cells varies partly due to a diurnal rythm and partly depending on the localization in the lobule[116, 210]. These normal variations are important to remember when interpreting the biopsy. When the morphological changes are pronounced and the specific staining is typical the differential diagnostic problem is small, but it is important in cases suspected of glycogen storage disease to reserve a part of the biopsy specimen for biochemical and histochemical analysis.

Additional morphological findings: Most biopsis from patients with glycogenosis show slight non-specific changes such as scattered focal necrosis and focal proliferation of Kupffer cells[226]. Usually the liver cells also contain fat droplets[218]. Fibrosis is sometimes to be found after longlasting disease.

In glycogenosis type I (v. Gierke's disease) development of cirrhosis is exceptionally rare but in, for instance, glycogenosis type IV cirrhosis of the liver nearly always arises[226].

For hepatocellular adenoma and carcinoma, see p. 194.

Occurence and significance: Inborn errors of metabolism known as glycogenosis have been described in at least eight different forms. Most of them involve the liver, but other organs, especially muscles, may also be affected. They are rare, the most common being v. Gierke's disease[226].

Accumulation of glycogen in liver cell tumors has diagnostic significance in the case of adenoma, and significance for typing in the case of liver-cell carcinoma.

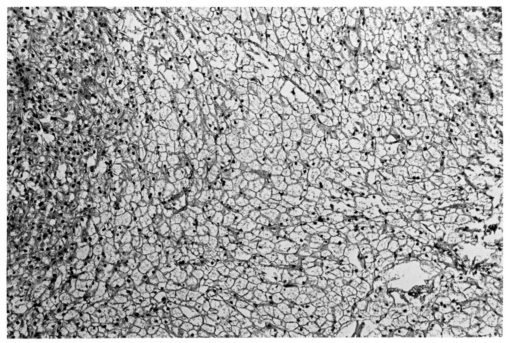

Fig. 100: Small magnification of a biopsy from a patient with glycogen storage disease. The cytoplasm of most of the liver cells is palely stained and the cell borders are distinct (Needle biopsy, H & E x 110).

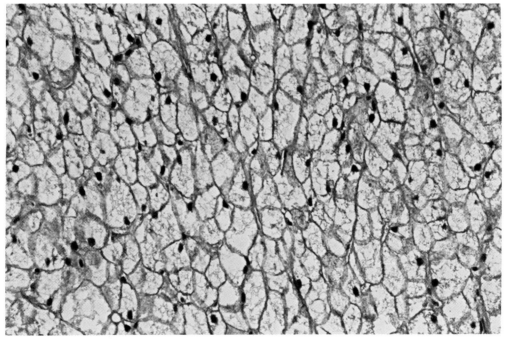

Fig. 101: Higher magnification of the same biopsy as Fig. 100. The cells have an appearance of plant cells. The nuclei are all small and many are located close to the cell border. No necrosis (Needle biopsy, H & E x 270).

PAS-positive, diastase resistant globules

Morphology: In H & E-stained sections these globules may be seen as circular or oval, well-demarcated bodies, 1 μm to more than 20 μm in diameter. They are eosinophilic and homogeneous, and are irregularly distributed in the cytoplasm of the liver cells. There is often a tendency to formation of small fissures between the globules and the adjacent cytoplasm (Fig. 102).

The affected liver cells are nearly always enlarged but usually not necrotic. The number of globules varies not only from cell to cell but also from area to area in the same biopsy and from biopsy to biopsy. In biopsies with preserved lobular architecture, the number of globules is as a rule highest in the periportal zone[337], and in cirrhosis most are localized in the peripheral parts of the parenchymal nodules[336]. Globules may be found extracellularly in areas with liver cell necrosis.

The globules stain intensely red by the PAS method[204]. They contain diastase-resistant glycoprotein and are for this reason most distinctly seen in sections stained with PAS after diastase digestion (Fig. 103). The globules are composed of alpha-l-antitrypsin and can be selectively stained immunohistochemically with immunofluorescent[39, 126] or immunoperoxidase techniques[303]. In the electron microscope an amorphous material in dilated rough endoplasmic reticulum is found[336].

Morphological diagnosis: The globules are very difficult to recognize at low magnifications in H & E-stained sections, and may easily be overlooked even at higher magnification especially when their number is small. On the other hand, they are very conspicuous in diastase-treated, PAS-stained sections, even under low power.

Differential diagnosis: Intracytoplasmic acidophilic inclusions in liver cells may be found in acute and chronic hepatitis as well as in post-hepatitic cirrhosis. Such inclusions are usually about the size of a liver cell nucleus and probably correspond to autophagic vacuoles[36]. They are PAS-negative.

Similar bodies may be seen in other conditions, e.g. steatosis. They are also PAS-negative.

So-called Mallory bodies have an irregular outline but may in early stages of their formation contain some globular structures[56]. They should not normally be confused with the globules in question (p. 110).

Acidophil bodies are transformed whole liver cells expelled from the liver cells plates and situated interstitially[36] (p. 80).

Additional morphologic findings: The presence of PAS-positive globules is regarded as a morphological expression of alpha-l-antitrypsin deficiency[132]. In some cases the liver tissue is otherwise quite normal and the number of globules is then usually small[337]. In many cases, however, the globules are associated with steatosis, fibrosis and/or cirrhosis[336].

Occurrence and significance: Publications showing the incidence of the globules in question in consecutive liver biopsy material are not available. Only few autopsy series have been investigated[303]. Positive globules have been noted in 3–6 per cent of the cases.

The change has a close relation to alpha-l-antitrypsin deficiency. Many patients with alpha-l-antitrypsin deficiency develop cirrhosis very early in life but the first signs of cirrhosis may make their debut later, possibly in the fifties or sixties[336, 252]. Cirrhosis of the liver is often associated with emphysema of the lung in adults, but each may be seen separately[204].

Diastase-resistant PAS-positive globules, which also are immunoreactive to alpha-l-antitrypsin but without relation to alpha-l-antitrypsin deficiency, may be demonstrated in focal lesions such as liver cell adenoma, liver cell carcinoma and focal nodular hyperplasia.

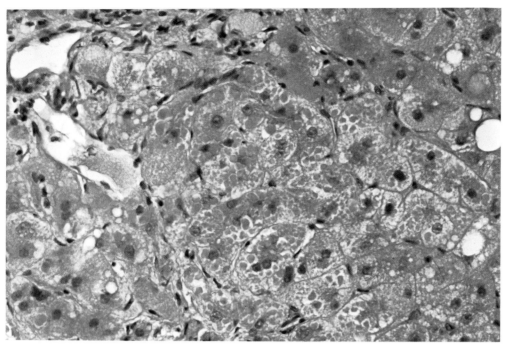

Fig. 102: Eosinophil globules of varying size in the cytoplasm of liver cells. In the upper left corner, part of a connective tissue area is seen. A few fat droplets are also visible (Needle biopsy, H & E x 270).

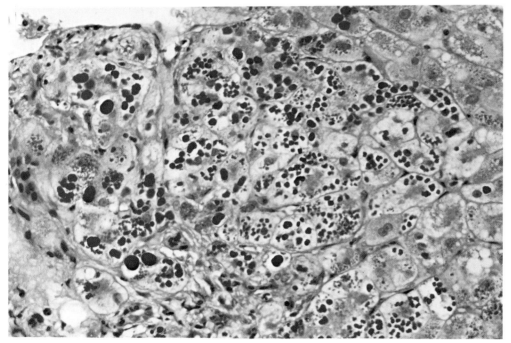

Fig. 103: Globules in the cytoplasm of liver cells. Same biopsy and same area as Fig. 102 (serial section). From a patient with alpha-l-antitrypsin deficiency with emphysema and cirrhosis (Needle biopsy, PAS after diastase x 270).

"Ground glass" – orcein positive

Morphology: The so-called "ground glass" change in liver cells usually involves most of the cytoplasm, which in H & E-stained sections appears light and finely granulated[346, 372]. The affected area of the cytoplasm appears more or less eosinophilic without or with only a minimal content of basophilic granules. The cells are nearly always somewhat enlarged but have preserved cell borders and nuclear structure.

The number of liver cells with "ground glass" change varies considerably from area to area in the individual biopsy and from biopsy to biopsy. In some cases only few cells are affected, while in others most cells are altered[151, 372].

On the basis of special stains, the "ground glass" change can be divided into two types; one type shows (probably on the basis of S=S bonds) a positive reaction with orcein staining[346, 372], whereas the other type gives a negative reaction[372] (see p. 118).

In the orcein-positive "ground glass" change the granules are very fine and of uniform size. The nucleus is as a rule located at one side of the cell close to the cell membrane, and there may be fissures around the ground glass area delimiting it from the rest of the cytoplasm (Fig. 104 & 105). This type of change is without characteristic location in the lobules or in cirrhotic nodules[372].

Ultrastructural investigations suggest that the common substrate for the two types is a marked hyperplasia of the smooth endoplasmic reticulum (SER) with ensuing displacement of other cytoplasmic components[152]. In the orcein-positive type, characteristic filaments are in addition found in the SER and this type also gives a conspicuous response to HB-antibody with immunofluorescence[302].

Morphological diagnosis: Only in cases with severe and widely distributed changes can the diagnosis be made at lower magnifications in H & E-stained sections[288].

By orcein[346] or aldehyde-fuchsin[346] staining the change is easier to diagnose because of the difference in color. The most specific demonstration is made by immunofluorescent[288, 302] and immunoperoxidase techniques[149] and good results may be obtained with paraffin-embedded material (Fig. 105).

Differential diagnosis: The lesion is easy to recognize in most cases when both H & E and orcein stains are available. Usually the orcein-negative ground glass change has a more or less different appearance when seen in H & E-stained sections, but in exceptional cases the difference is minimal (p. 118).

Additional morphological findings: Orcein-positive "ground glass" change is so far only described in HB_SAg-positive patients. It is most frequently found in so-called healthy carriers of HB_SAg whose biopsies either show a normal picture or slight non-specific changes[152]. Many healthy carriers have widely distributed "ground glass" change. Orcein positive "ground glass" change is moreover seen (usually only in scattered liver cells) in chronic persistent and chronic aggressive hepatitis, in cirrhosis, and in acute viral hepatitis with signs of chronicity[151], whereas is has not been demonstrated in biopsies exhibiting changes of acute viral hepatitis without signs of chronicity.

Occurrence and significance: Orcein-positive "ground glass" change occurs in healthy HB_SAg carriers (often more than 50 per cent of the cases)[152] and in some HB_SAg-positive patients with longstanding acute hepatitis, chronic hepatitis, or cirrhosis[151].

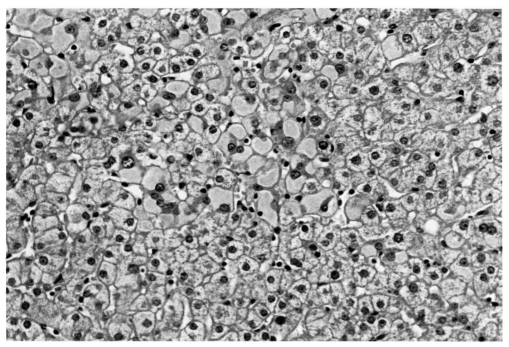

Fig. 104: Widely distributed "ground-glass" change with many enlarged liver cells with a cytoplasm which appears eosinophilic, light and finely granular. In most instances the nuclei are dislocated (Needle biopsy, H & E x 270).

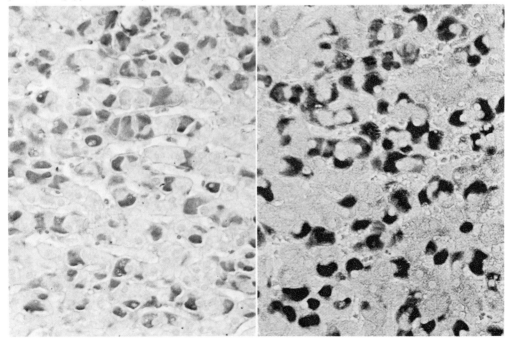

Fig. 105: Left. Widely distributed orcein-positive "ground-glass" change (orcein). Right. Same lesion demonstrated with immunoperoxidase. From a so-called healthy carrier. Same biopsy as Fig. 104 (Needle biopsy x 270).

"Ground glass" - orcein negative

Morphology: Orcein-negative "ground glass" change can – as is the case for the orcein-positive form – comprise larger or smaller parts of the liver cell cytoplasm, but in general it involves all the cytoplasm[372]. Compared with the positive form the granules are somewhat coarser and more irregular in size, and as a rule the eosinophilia is slightly less pronounced (Fig. 106). Fissures can only exceptionally be demonstrated. The nuclei are rarely dislocated and then usually only to a slight degree. The cytoplasmic change does not give a positive reaction with orcein or aldehyde-fuchsin[372].

In most cases accumulation of basophilic material at the biliary poles of the cells or around the nucleus is characteristic.

The changes are usually widespread, comprising many adjoining cells. Quite often there is a zonal preponderance, as a rule centrilobular but occasionally periportal.

Morphological diagnosis: The changes are best seen in H & E-stained sections, and in our experience no special staining has significant diagnostic importance. Severe and widespread changes are easily found at lower magnifications but slighter changers necessitate a closer view.

Differential diagnosis: It is usually possible on H & E-stained sections to distiguish the orcein-negative from the orcein-positive form as the orcein-negative "ground glass" change has a more irregular granularity often associated with canalicular accumulation of basophilic material, is less well demarcated, and involves larger groups of cells often with zonal distribution[372].

In rare cases the orcein-negative changes as seen for instance in glycogenosis IV and in myoclonal epilepsy may look very similar to the orcein-positive form on H & E.

Another important differential diagnosis is the type of artefact sometimes seen in the marginal portions of a biopsy and characterized by a strong eosinophilia of the liver cells[212]. If a biopsy shows artefacts of this kind, it is consequently only possible to diagnose the lesion in areas with well-preserved liver cells, i.e. the central part of the specimen.

Additional morphological findings: Orceinnegative "ground glass" appearance may be found in drug-induced and toxic liver injury. This change has been called induction or adaption[78], in the literature, and is seen with high frequency after, for example, barbiturates[356] and sometimes chlorpromazine or alcohol[308]. Thus the "ground glass" change may be seen together with other drug-induced or toxic liver changes, for instance non-specific reactive hepatitis, steatosis and alcoholic hepatitis and accumulation of lipofuscin and lipofuscin-like pigment.

Occurrence and significance: We have found this form of "ground glass" change in approximately 5 per cent of our biopsies. The change is usually a light microscopic expression of the influence of inducing agents, that is substances which are capable of increasing the amount of enzymes by adaptation[231]. Most common are derivatives of benzodiapam (Librium, Diazepam, Valium, Stesolid etc.), barbiturates, phenylbutazone, diphenylhydantoin, antituberculous drugs and cyclophosphamide. In addition alcohol may act as an inducing agent and similar changes are described in both degenerative and regenerative liver cell lesions as well as in hepatocellular carcinoma. Sometimes no cause for the lesion can be found (Fig. 107).

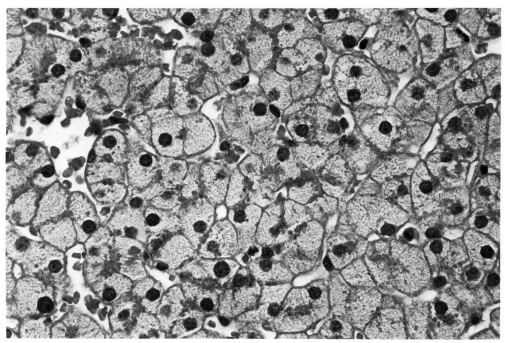

Fig. 106: Widely distributed orcein-negative "ground-glass" change. All the liver cells are enlarged with weakly stained, diffusely granular cytoplasm. In some of the cells basophilic granules are visible around bile canaliculi. Chronic alcoholism (Needle biopsy, H & E x 400).

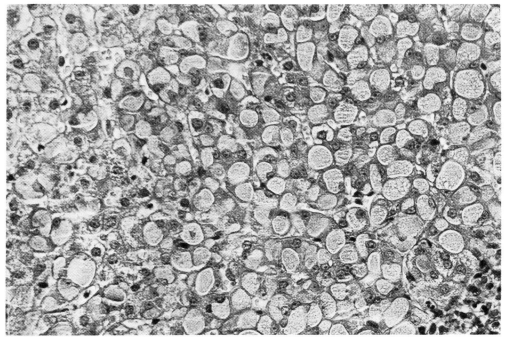

Fig. 107: Widely distributed "ground-glass" change. The picture is very similar to the orcein-positive "ground-glass" type but orcein is negative. Middle-aged female, previously alcoholic; no clinical signs of myoclonal epilepsia (Needle biopsy, H & E x 270).

Siderosis

Morphology: By siderosis is understood the presence of stainable iron in the liver tissue[327i]. It is most commonly found in liver cells and/or Kupffer cells. Iron is bound in the cells as hemosiderin which is a complex with variable quantities of carbohydrates, proteins and iron[396]. In tissue sections, hemosiderin can be seen as golden yellow granules. The iron is in a trivalent state and gives a positive Prussian blue reaction. The siderosis of liver cells is virtually always periportal in localization in non-cirrhotic tissue and ranges from a few granules to a massive overload with blurring of cellular details[328]. The iron deposition in liver cells may be found in otherwise normal liver parenchyma[328] (Fig. 108 & 109), superimposed on a pre-existing cirrhosis[180], or preceding the development of cirrhosis as in hemochromatosis[147].

In hemochromatosis there is massive iron deposition in the liver cells in connection with tissue damage as seen by focal necrosis, periportal and parenchymal fibrosis and development of cirrhosis[147]. Pigment is also found in Kupffer cells, connective tissue and bile duct epithelium[147].

Iron-containing pigment in Kupffer cells only is most typically seen in acute hepatitis[265, 289] (see p. 174).

Morphological diagnosis: Iron can be recognized in H & E-stained sections but reliable identification of small amounts and safe differentiation from lipofuscin and ceroid requires specific staining for iron. Perls' staining procedure[260] is recommended as a routine on all biopsies. Serial sections stained for reticulin and collagen fibers may be necessary in order to identify a possible increase in connective tissue.

Differential diagnosis: Differentiation between cirrhosis in patients with hemochromatosis and cirrhosis accompanied by liver cell siderosis may be difficult. Examination of earlier biopsies of such patients may show that in cirrhosis with superimposed hemosiderosis the cirrhosis has preceded the iron deposition, whereas the reverse is the case in hemochromatosis. The iron in septa is a feature of some significance[180]. Abundance of iron-containing histiocytes in the septa indicates that cirrhosis developed at a time when iron excess was present in the liver. Their absence implies that siderosis has developed after cirrhosis was fully established.

Additional morphological findings: Liver cell siderosis is particularly common in chronic alcoholics[66] and is often associated with fatty change, alcoholic hepatitis and cirrhosis. In hemochromatosis a cirrhosis with a relatively characteristic jigsaw puzzle-like pattern is usual[180].

Occurrence and significance: Iron excess of varying degrees is common in patients with cirrhosis[21]. The iron may be confined to the liver or it may be found in the liver and in parenchymal cells of other organs. When the iron load is heavy the condition resembles, and may be erroneously diagnosed as, idiopathic hemochromatosis.

Siderosis is common in anemia, especially in certain types of refractory anemias both acquired and congenital[179]. While in the acquired types tissue damage is rare and, if present, usually mild, those with congenital defects often display advanced cirrhosis.

Overload resulting from increased dietary intake is seen as an iatrogenic disorder in patients treated with iron and in alcoholics due to iron in alcoholic beverages[102]. Tissue damage and cirrhosis occur in a small but significant number of patients.

Iron overload has been implicated in the pathogenesis of porphyria cutanea tarda, but the exact role of iron is not established[26].

About 50 per cent of our biopsies from patients with acute hepatitis show iron containing pigment in Kupffer cells and portal macrophages[265].

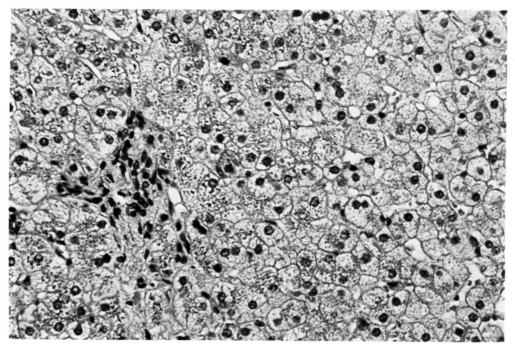

Fig. 108: Part of liver lobule with a portal tract at the left. A great number of brown granules of varying size is seen in the liver cells, especially in the periportal part of the lobule (Needle biopsy, H & E x 270).

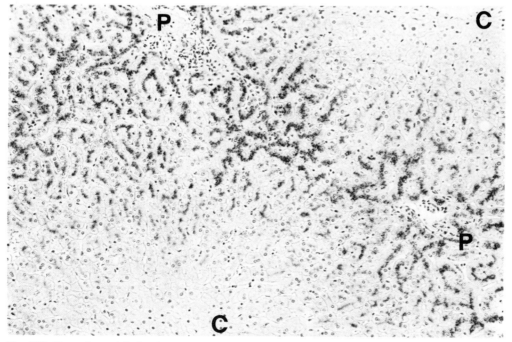

Fig. 109: Part of two lobules from the same biopsy as Fig. 108. The amount of pigment is larger in the liver cells around the portal tracts (P) than around the central veins (C). From a patient with siderosis (Needle biopsy, Perls' stain for iron x 110).

Lipofuscin and lipofuscin-like pigment

Morphology: Lipofuscin appears in the cytoplasm of the liver cells as fine brown granules arranged in small clumps near the bile canaliculi. It is a pigment which contains some fatty material, allowing it to be stained with certain fat stains[217]. Ultrastructural and histochemical investigations have shown that this pigment is normally formed and contained by the lysosomes[128]. The granules are approximately 1 μm in diameter, and in younger persons are most abundant in the central parts of the lobules, around the central veins. The amount of lipofuscin increases with age, and it is seen in high concentration especially in atrophic livers. The pigment has been called "wear and tear" product[287]. In older persons lipofuscin is seen not only in liver cells around the central veins, but also in periportal cells.

Increased lipofuscin in liver cells is seen following prolonged intake of some drugs, including phenacetin and chlorpromazine[148], and when the amount of pigment is plentiful the pericanalicular location is no longer evident. In passive congestion with atrophy of liver cells the amount of lipofuscin is also increased[342]. In Wilson's disease liver cell lipofuscin is sometimes abundant[323], whereas the amount is decreased in areas of proliferating liver cells. In liver cell adenomas areas with strongly pigmented cells may be seen (Fig. 110).

The Dubin-Johnson syndrome[107] is characterized by the presence of large amounts of a yellow-brown or black pigment in otherwise normal liver cells. Macroscopically the liver is black or very dark brown. The pigment is most pronounced in the central parts of the lobules and is often seen also in Kupffer cells. The granules are larger, darker and show greater variation in size than normal lipofuscin (Fig. 111) but occupy a similar pericanalicular site in the cell. Histochemical stains do not distinguish with certainty between the two kinds of pigment but it is probable that the Dubin-Johnson pigment has a melanin-like composition[13].

Morphological diagnosis: Normal lipofuscin is best recognized in H & E-stained sections or in sections stained for iron by Perls' method[260]. The recognition of small changes in the amount of pigment may be difficult because of normal variation, and demands some experience. The pigment is PAS-positive to a variable degree, and acid fast[277]. The most sensitive method is, however, the ferric ferricyanide method.

The recognition of Dubin-Johnson pigment is usually easy on the basis of the morphological characteristics and the dark color of the biopsy macroscopically[107].

Differential diagnosis: Lipofuscin may be difficult to distinguish from intracellular granules of bile, but the latter are nearly always accompanied by bile plugs in the canaliculi. In hemosiderosis the lipofuscin pigment may be masked by the iron which occupies the same intracellular sites. In these cases Perls' stain may be helpful.

Additional morphological findings: Increased lipofuscin following intake of phenacetin or chlorpromazine[148] is sometimes accompanied by centrilobular cholestasis. When cholestasis is present varying degrees of portal and parenchymal inflammation are often demonstrable, and cases with a histological picture of acute hepatitis, usually mild, have also been reported. In Wilson's disease the excess lipofuscin is seen together with accumulation of copper and signs of progressive liver cell destruction[323].

The Dubin-Johnson pigment is characteristically found in otherwise normal liver and there is no cholestasis[107].

Occurrence and significance: Slight changes in the amount of lipofuscin are of no diagnostic significance, whereas an appreciable increase is most commonly found in relation to cachetic conditions or prolonged intake of drugs[148]. The Dubin-Johnson pigment is diagnostic for this disease.

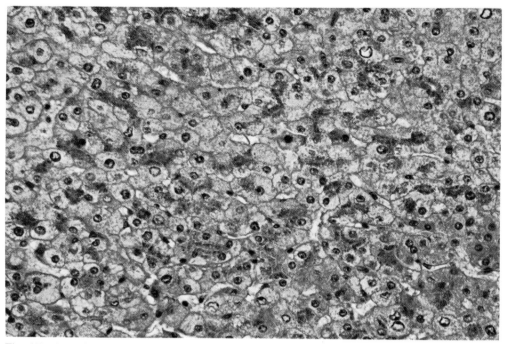

Fig. 110: Area from a hepatocellular adenoma. There is a pronounced hyperpigmentation with clusters of light brown, fine granules in the cells. The granules are seen mainly around the bile canaliculi (Surgical biopsy, H & E x 270).

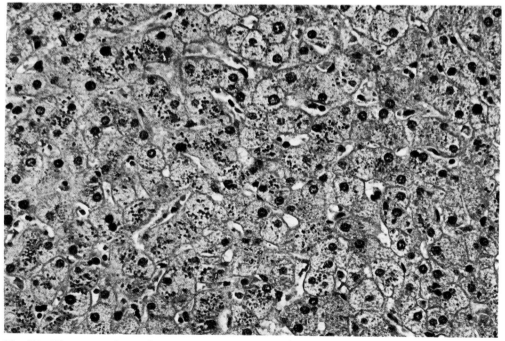

Fig. 111: Liver parenchyma from a patient with the Dubin-Johnson syndrome. There are many dark brown granules diffusely distributed in the cytoplasm of the liver cells. The granules are of varying size, most often large (Needle biopsy, H & E x 270).

Copper accumulation

Morphology: Normally the liver tissue contains only very small amounts of copper (less than 100 µg/g dry weight) and it is present diffusely in the cytoplasm[324]. Essential quantitative and qualitative alterations are necessary before the copper can be demonstrated histochemically. It is only possible in cases where the copper is condensed in the lysosomal granules[323]. The lysosomes have a diameter of 0.5–5 µm and are localized around the nuclei, and the copper accumulation is most often found in periportal hepatocytes. Often the copper can be seen only focally and in few liver cells in relation to a single or a few portal tracts. In cases with severe accumulation the distribution may be more diffuse[347].

Copper can be demonstrated histochemically by a series of methods[205]. In our experience the best combination of sensitivity and specificity is achieved with rubeanic acid, which gives the granules a green-black or black color (Fig. 112) or with dimethylaminobenzylidine-rhodanine (DMABR) which gives a distinct red color.

The same granules are stained brown-black with orcein (Fig. 113) and red with PAS possibly because of the free sulphhydryl groups in the copper binding protein metallothionin[313].

Morphological diagnosis: Orcein staining is the most suitable method for screening for the presence of copper[313]. The metal itself is more specifically demonstrated with rubeanic acid or DMABR. H & E-stained sections are unsuitable for the demonstration of copper.

Differential diagnosis: In addition to metallothionin, elastin and HB_SAg, orcein stains ceroid in Kupffer cells and portal macrophages[372]. In a minority of cases there may be differential diagnostic problems with respect to ceroid but the copper staining is negative.

Rubeanic acid and DMABR sometimes give weak staining of iron containing granules. This is an exception and may possibly be explained by the mutual presence of both metals. Both stains may in addition react with other metals which is, however, currently of no practical value in liver biopsy diagnosis.

Additional morphological findings: Since copper containing granules particularly occur in Wilson's disease[325] and in primary biliary cirrhosis[162, 347], morphological changes as found in these diseases are often present. Copper-containing granules may also be seen in other conditions especially in relation to longstanding cholestasis, for instance in secondary biliary cirrhosis[314].

Occurrence and significance: Histochemically demonstrable copper is found in largest amounts in Wilson's disease and in primary biliary cirrhosis and may in such cases be of importance for the diagnosis, since the other morphological changes in these conditions are not uncommonly non-specific. The presence of copper may in particular be important for the differential diagnosis between primary biliary cirrhosis and chronic aggressive hepatitis.

Copper may in addition be found in some cases of alcoholic liver disease with fibrosis[305] or cirrhosis and to a lesser degree also in other forms of cirrhosis[162]. Finally, copper accumulation may, as indicated above, be seen in cases with longstanding cholestasis[314].

By biochemical and other methods large amounts of copper – especially in Wilson's disease – have been demonstrated in the liver tissue even in cases where it has been impossible to demonstrate copper histochemically[200]. This discrepancy is possibly due to an increase in the diffusely dispersed copper, since it is probable that the histochemical reactions are only positive when appreciable concentrations, such as are found in lysosomes, are present.

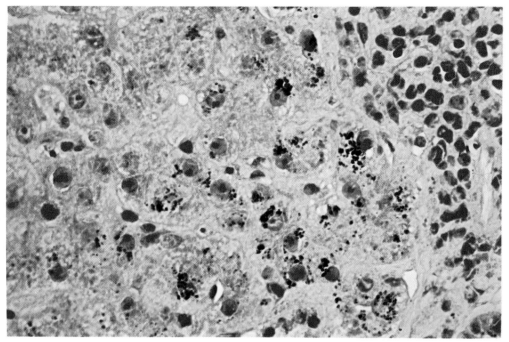

Fig. 112: Peripheral part of a lobule with part of adjacent portal tract (right). Black granules of different sizes are seen in the cytoplasm of the liver cells (Needle biopsy, rubeanic acid x 400).

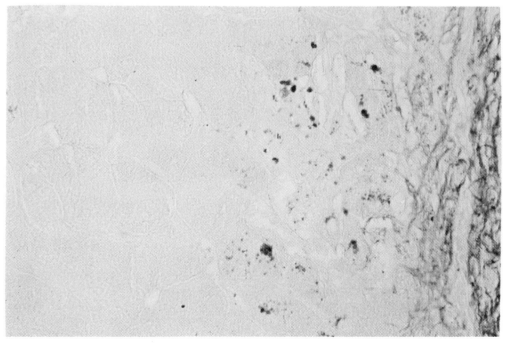

Fig. 113: Same part of the lobule and adjacent portal tract (right) as shown in Fig. 112. Brownish granules are seen in the periportal parenchyma but cellular details are inconspicuous (Needle biopsy, orcein x 400).

Other accumulations

Morphology: Hepatocellular *bile pigment* occurs as yellow-green or brown granules in the cytoplasm and is usually associated with canalicular bile plugs. The size of the granules varies considerably. They are most often found in the centrilobular zones and in the pericanalicular parts of the cells (Fig. 114), but they may occur more diffusely in both the lobules and in the cytoplasm.

Uroporphyrin may, when the liver is affected in porphyria cutanea tarda, be demonstrated in both liver cells and in macrophages[209]. Uroporphyrin has a strong autofluorescence, which is pink to orange-red, and which is most distinct in ultraviolet light. The substance is not a pigment and cannot be seen in ordinary light. On fixation the structure is altered and the fluorescence disappears.

In some biopsies, mainly from alcoholics, the cytoplasm of non-necrotic hepatocytes contains one or more round or elongated homogeneous *hyaline bodies* of regular outline[165] (Fig. 115). These cytoplasmic hyaline inclusions are different from Mallory bodies and under the electron microscope they appear as megamitochondria.

Morphological diagnosis: Bile pigment in the cytoplasm of the liver cells can be recognized in H & E-stained sections but demonstration is easier and safer in sections stained for iron or with the van Gieson stain.

In cases with large amounts of uroporphyrin the fluorescence can be visualized in ultraviolet light on the whole, unfixed biopsy cylinder. The safest method, however, is investigation of frozen sections under the UV-microscope[209].

The hyaline inclusions in alcoholics stain pink with eosin and red with trichrome.

Differential diagnosis: Intracellular granules of bile may be difficult to distinguish from lipofuscin, but the usual presence of bile thrombi in the canaliculi may be helpful. Both bile pigment and lipofuscin may be positive with PAS staining, but as distinct from lipofuscin, bile pigment gives no reaction by the long Ziehl-Neelsen method.

Uroporphyrin has such a characteristic red color in autofluorescence that it should not be confused with any other substance[209].

The hyaline inclusions in question are PAS-negative and are therefore easily distinguished from globular deposits in patients with alpha-l-antitrypsin deficiency which are diastase – PAS-positive.

Additional morphological findings: Bile pigment in hepatocytes is nearly always found together with bile thrombi in canaliculi, and all the changes in parenchyma and portal tracts described in connection with cholestasis (p. 184) may be found.

Accumulation of uroporphyrin in the liver is seen in porphyria cutanea tarda. Many of these patients are alcoholics and among other things steatosis, siderosis, fibrosis and cirrhosis may be present[26].

The megamitochondria are most often seen in alcoholics and all the changes described in the alcoholic liver may be found.

Occurrence and significance: Bile droplets within hepatocytes are usually associated with canalicular bile plugs. Occurrence and significance ase discussed on p. 184.

The presence of uroporphyrin is diagnostic for porphyria cutanea tarda. Many such cases are subclinical and routine investigation of liver biopsies under ultraviolet light is recommended.

The significance of the megamitochondria is at present not known.

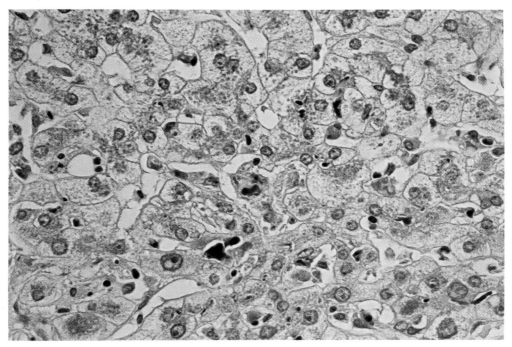

Fig. 114: Part of lobule from a patient with acute hepatitis with slight parenchymal damage and severe cholestasis. In addition to bile plugs in Kupffer cells and between liver cells, there are tiny granules in the cytoplasm (Needle biopsy, van Gieson x 270).

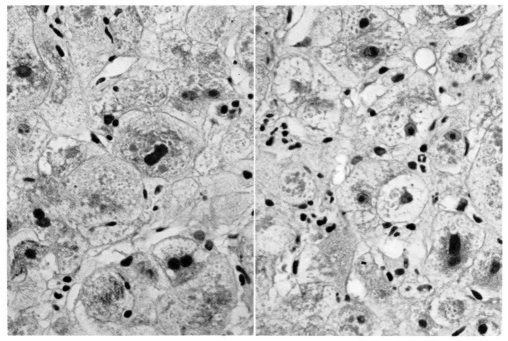

Fig. 115: Left. In the center is an enlarged liver cell with two eosinophilic globules. Right. Another area with many similar but smaller globules. The globules are all PAS-negative. From a chronic alcoholic (Needle biopsy, H & E x 400).

Normal

Morphology: The liver cell plates are exposed on both sides to the blood moving from the portal tracts to the central veins. The blood flows in the sinusoids[237], which are radially arranged around the central veins. There are many intercommunications between the sinusoids through fenestrations in the liver cell plates, and the sinusoidal system thus forms an extended labyrinthine vessel bed.

The sinusoids are slightly irregular in shape, and the lumen is normally narrow and empty in biopsy specimens, but sometimes areas with many erythrocytes and a few scattered white corpuscles may be found (Fig. 116 & 117). Exceptionally, a single bone-marrow cell, e.g. a megakarocyte, is present in an otherwise normal biopsy. The lining cells of the sinusoids[12], often named the littoral cells of the liver, form a flat layer on the supporting reticulin fibers contained in the space of Disse. Two types of lining cells are recognized, endothelial cells and Kupffer cells[193, 386]. Endothelial cells are the most common and have small, dark nuclei. The cytoplasm is scanty and attenuated to form thin sheets with perforations arranged in small groups (sieve plates)[246]. These cells loosely overlap each other like roof shingles, leaving open gaps between them[392]. Kupffer cells are larger, with more cytoplasm and larger nuclei, often with prominent nucleoli. Kupffer cells may contain phagocytic material in the cytoplasm[193] and sometimes these cells may be found as bridging cells, sitting spider-like across the spaces[80]. It is probable that the Kupffer cells can bulge into the lumen of a sinusoids, obliterating it in part or entirely and thereby playing a role in regulating the sinusoidal blood flow[312].

Between the lining cells and the liver cells there is a perivascular space, the space of Disse[130]. This is not visible under the light microscope but clearly demonstrable electronmicroscopically. The liver cells show large numbers of microvilli, and a constant striking feature is the occurrence of predominantly longitudinally orientated reticulin fibers[246] (p. 150). In the space of Disse scattered lipocytes (Ito cells) are found[44, 169] which are very similar to fibroblasts[363] but have fat vacuoles in their cytoplasm. The Ito cells may sometimes be suspected lightmicroscopically by their dark nuclei and localization, but identification is not easy and not always convincing.

Morphological diagnosis: The diagnosis of normal sinusoids is usually easy. Both low and high magnifications should be used and H & E as well as stains for reticulin and collagen fibers are necessary. The presence of abnormal pigment must be excluded.

Differential diagnosis: The lumen of normal sinusoids is as a rule narrow, although some variation may be found. Broad sinusoids in a specimen are probably normal when the liver cell plates show no atrophy. Small amounts of pigment are easily overlooked.

Areas with normal sinusoids are often found in cirrhotic livers. In the majority of these cases multiple sections disclose abnormal sinusoids with, for instance, fibrosis or other abnormalities such as thickened liver cell plates.

Additional morphological findings: Normal sinusoids in all areas of a biopsy are as a rule seen only in otherwise normal liver tissue or in liver tissue with slight changes, for instance steatosis or siderosis.

Occurrence and significance: Only relatively few of our biopsies show normal sinusoids in all parts since even small parenchymal changes such as a focal liver cell necrosis affect the sinusoids. Completely normal sinusoids in a large, well-processed biopsy excludes many diagnoses such as acute hepatitis, chronic aggressive hepatitis, and cirrhosis.

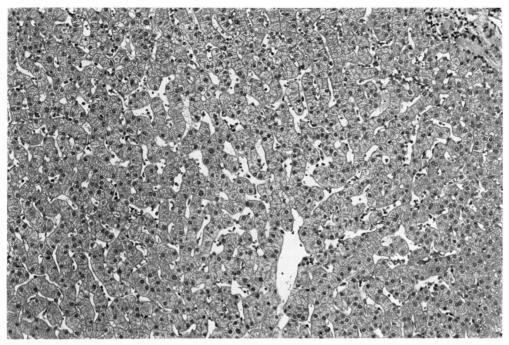

Fig. 116: Part of normal lobule with a central vein in the lower middle third and a small part of a portal tract in the upper right corner. A few of the sinusoids contain some erythrocytes (Needle biopsy, H & E x 110).

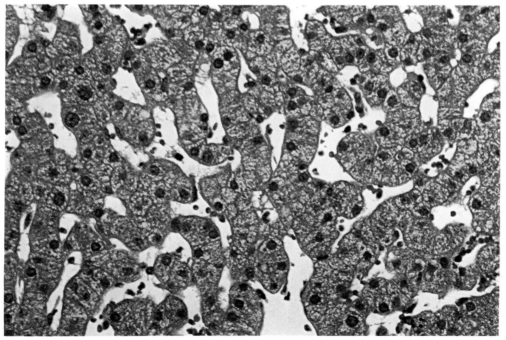

Fig. 117: Part of centrilobular area from the same liver lobule as Fig. 116. The sinusoids are of normal width and both lining cells and erythrocytes are to be found. There is no atrophy of the liver cells plates (Needle biopsy, H & E x 270).

Dilatation

Morphology: Dilatation of the sinusoids may be of all degrees and is accompanied by a corresponding narrowing of the liver cell plates. The dilated sinusoids have preserved lining cells and may contain varying amounts of blood corpuscles, although in most biopsies many appear empty.

In liver tissue with preserved lobular architecture the dilatation is most common in the centrilobular zone (Fig. 118) possibly with involvement of the intermediate zone[295]. Periportal sinusoidal dilatation, also with a tendency to affect the intermediate zone, has also been described (Fig. 119)[395]. More localized and irregularly distributed dilatation may be found for instance in cirrhosis, liver cell adenomas (Fig. 89), and liver cell carcinomas. Transitions between sinusoidal dilatation and peliosis[399] are sometimes seen.

Morphological diagnosis: The diagnosis is made at low magnifications on H & E-stained sections. An important feature is the accompanying atrophy of the liver cells and the usually zonal distribution.

Differential diagnosis: The histological picture is nearly always characteristic, and there are only two differential diagnostic problems. The first is the differentiation between the mildest changes and normal liver (p. 128), and the second is an artefact with increased distance between some of the liver cell plates. This latter change is found in the peripheral part of the biopsy and is possibly caused by an excessive negative pressure during the performance of the biopsy. It is more commonly found with the use of the Vim-Silverman needle than with the Menghini needle, and is more frequent in small and fragmented biopsies. The artefact is often accompanied by other artefacts, such as condensation, increased eosinophilia and positive iron staining of the liver cells in the same area[178]. Atrophy of the liver plates is absent.

Additional morphological findings: Centrilobular sinusoidal dilation also often involves the intermediate zone and is here sometimes associated with a slight degree of steatosis[295]. Centrilobular confluent necrosis and conspicuous cholestasis is also to be found in some cases, and some degree of centrilobular fibrosis may develop in long-standing conditions.

Periportal sinusoidal dilatation is accompanied by slight portal and periportal infiltration with lymphocytes and histiocytes. The portal tracts are otherwise normal. The centrilobular zone is virtually unaffected except that slight cholestasis may be present[395].

The focal and more irregularly distributed dilatation may be found in some cases of cirrhosis, liver cell adenomas and carcinomas, and consequently, one may find the other changes of these diseases (chapter III).

Occurrence and significance: Centrilobular sinusoidal dilatation is most often found in patients with increased hepatic venous pressure caused by right ventricular failure or exceptionally by thrombus or tumor[37]. There are, however, patients in whom no obvious cause can be demonstrated[295]. They usually suffer from chronic diseases (malignant disease, connective tissue disease), and most have increased levels of serum gamma globulins and low serum albumin.

Periportal sinusoidal dilatation is unusual and so far only observed in female patients in the fertile age on long-term treatment with contraceptive steroids[395]. Clinically these patients developed moderate hepatomegaly and possibly slight jaundice. The course of the disease seems to be benign.

In peliosis multiple blood-filled spaces with or without lining epithelium is present[399]. It may be found in a variety of diseases, for instance tuberculosis, or follow noxious substances such as polyvinyl chloride. The etiology is unknown but some may develop from sinusoidal dilatation after prolonged administration of anabolic or contraceptive steroids.

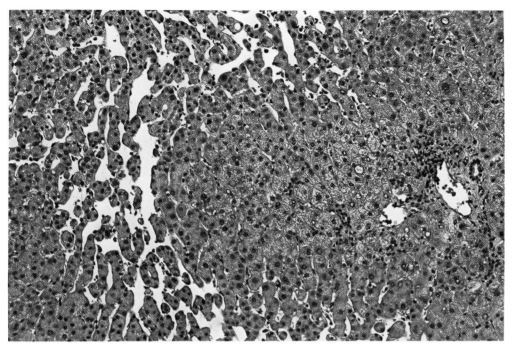

Fig. 118: Part of liver lobule with a portal tract to the right and a central vein area to the left. In the latter sinusoidal dilatation with some atrophy of the liver cell plates is unmistakable. Right-sided heart failure (Needle biopsy, H & E x 110).

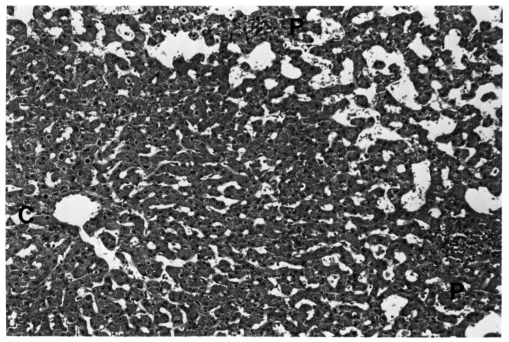

Fig. 119: Part of a liver lobule with a centrel vein (C) and two portal tracts (P). There are pronounced sinusoidal dilatation and atrophy of the liver cell plates in the periportal region. Hepatomegaly following intake of contraceptive pills (Needle biopsy, H & E 110).

Lining cell prominence and proliferation

Morphology: The sinusoidal lining cells may be enlarged (lining cell prominence) or increased in number (lining cell proliferation). The two changes are most commonly found together but may be demonstrated separately.

Lining cell prominence may include both endothelial cells and Kupffer cells[10]. The nuclei are enlarged and darker than normal, and the change is usually seen without liver cell necrosis (Fig. 120). The changes may involve whole lobules or, more commonly parts of lobules. In the more diffuse form of lining cell prominence rows of closely set nuclei are conspicuous along the sinusoidal border.

Lining cell proliferation particularly affects the Kupffer cells[10, 22]. It is not clear whether this proliferation is caused by mitotic activity or whether the enhanced number of cells is a consequence of maturation of monocytes[379]. The lesion is usually localized (Fig. 121) but may be diffuse. Even slight focal proliferation is usually found in connection with focal liver cell necrosis. This close relation between liver cell necrosis and lining cell proliferation is demonstrable by means of serial sections. Lymphocytes and sometimes also plasma cells, neutrophils and eosinophils may be found. The foci vary in extent but are most often of the order of two to five liver cells.

Morphological diagnosis: As previously pointed out, the normal sinusoidal lining cells vary in size, and scattered cells contain normally small amounts of ceroid. It therefore calls for some experience to distinguish slight prominence from the normal state.

Focal proliferation is easily recognized and diagnosed in H & E-stained sections even at low magnification. Special staining procedures are necessary for closer identification of pigment (p. 134).

Differential diagnosis: Lining cell prominence and proliferation hardly ever cause differential diagnostic problems. Well-demarcated focal proliferation may sometimes have a granulomatous appearance. Serial sections are helpful.

Additional morpholigical findings: Prominence and proliferation of sinusoidal lining cells occur in varying degrees together with many different parenchymal and portal changes.

Occurrence and significance: Prominence and proliferation of the sinusoidal lining cells are to be found in the great majority of biopsies, and since these changes are seen in so many different diseases, their presence is of only slight diagnostic significance. For pigments and other accumulations see p. 134 and p. 136.

The presence of conspicuous diffuse prominence is very characteristic for infectious mononucleosis[17, 387]. In addition one most often finds focal lining cell proliferation and focal liver cell necrosis although usually to a slight degree. Diffuse prominence may in addition be found in some cases of chronic hepatitis and cirrhosis as well as in gastrointestinal diseases. More continuous proliferations of atypical sinusoidal lining cells may be seen as a precursor stage to hemangiosarcoma (p. 196).

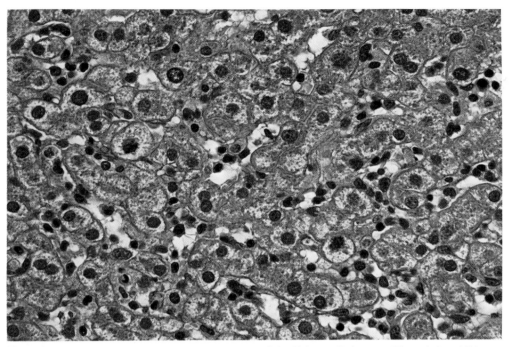

Fig. 120: In many sinusoids a marked prominence of the lining cells is seen. There is in addition a slight lining cell proliferation. Two liver cells (middle left and lower right) show mitosis. Infectious mononucleosis (Needle biopsy, H & E x 270).

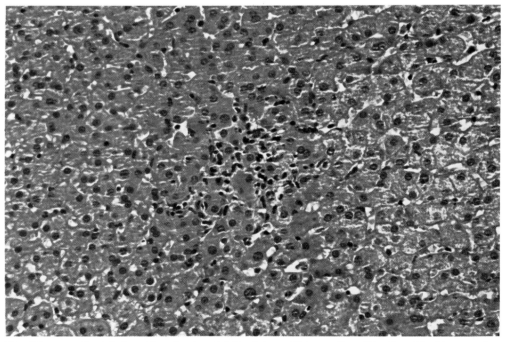

Fig. 121: Part of a lobule with a focal and fairly intense lining cell proliferation. Doubt may arise as to whether one or a few liver cells are necrotic or missing. Serial sections made it probable that there is no liver cell necrosis (Needle biopsy, H & E x 110).

Lining cells, pigment

Morphology: The most commonly found pigments in the sinusoidal lining cells are, as in the portal tracts, ceroid and iron.

Normally Kupffer cells may contain small amounts of ceroid; pathologically increased quantities are usually seen in biopsies with focal proliferation. It is generally accepted that both ceroid and iron, which are first seen in the Kupffer cells, are later transported to the portal tracts[28, 96].

Ceroid is seen as fine golden brown granules in the Kupffer cells. It may be found in solitary, enlarged cells but most often occurs in smaller or larger groups of proliferating cells. It is assumed that ceroid is formed in the Kupffer cells from phagocytized lipofuscin liberated by liver cell necrosis[28, 96].

Iron is found as fine, dark brown granules often together with ceroid and with a similar distribution[265]. Both types of pigments may be seen in all areas of the lobules.

Bile pigment is seen as small clumps inside the Kupffer cells[327c]. These have most often proliferated and formed smaller or larger groups. In H & E-stained sections the bile pigment is usually green but in older cases the color is brownish (Fig. 122).

Carbon, thorotrast[334] and *malarial*[110] pigment are sometimes seen in Kupffer cells, and have the same appearance as in portal histiocytes (p. 58).

Morphological diagnosis: As mentioned in connection with pigments in portal histiocytes, it is recommended that special stain should be used in order to identify and differentiate small amounts. We recommand PAS after disastase for ceroid (Fig. 123) and Perls' stain for iron. The latter offers in addition a good method for the identification of bile pigment.

Differential diagnosis: For the differentiation between ceroid and iron in Kupffer cells, see above. The bile pigment is green to brownish on H & E and appears green in van Gieson's- and Perls'-stained sections.

Additional morphological findings: The deposition of different forms of pigment in a few, isolated Kupffer cells may be found in otherwise normal liver tissue. Increased quantities of ceroid and iron in Kupffer cells are a phenomenon most often seen in connection with acute[29] and chronic hepatitis[58].

Bile in Kupffer cells may be demonstrated in all forms of cholestasis provided that it has lasted for some time[327b]. Consequently, bile in Kupffer cells may be present, for instance in large duct obstruction, acute viral hepatitis and primary biliary cirrhosis.

Occurrence and significance: Solitary Kupffer cells containing ceroid are usually seen in connection with focal necrosis. Smaller or larger groups of proliferating Kupffer cells with ceroid are always seen in acute hepatitis[29, 265], first with centrilobular distribution but later also in the peripheral parts of the lobules.

Isolated Kupffer cells containing iron are seen in hemosiderosis[147] and hemolytic conditions[179]. Proliferating Kupffer cells with iron positive pigment are found in approximately half the cases of acute hepatitis[265], mainly in the later stages.

Carbon, thorotrast and malarial pigment are rare and usually found together with similar pigments in portal histiocytes (p. 58).

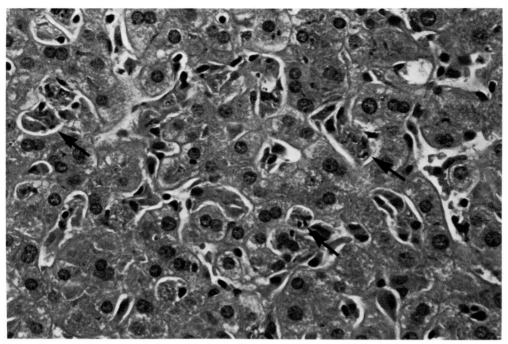

Fig. 122: Bile pigment in Kupffer cells. Many Kupffer cells are swollen and in the cytoplasm many green or brownish-green plugs of varying size are seen (arrows). Large duct obstruction and cholestasis for 2 weeks (Needle biopsy, H & E x 400).

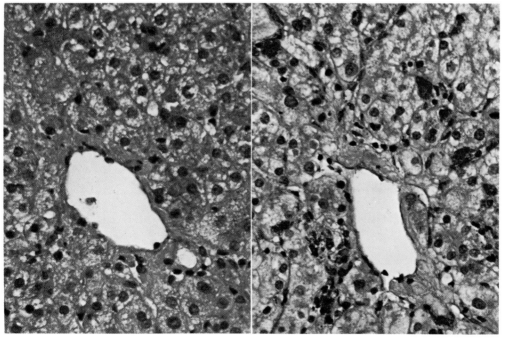

Fig. 123: From a patient with acute hepatitis. Swollen Kupffer cells in relation to focal liver cell necrosis are seen. Left. Ceroid pigment is brownish, inconspicuous (H & E). Right. The pigment is red, prominent (PAS after diastase) (Needle biopsy x 270).

Lining cells, accumulations

Morphology: In *Gaucher's disease*[133, 332] scattered Gaucher cells probably derived from Kupffer cells are seen throughout the parenchyma (Fig. 124). The Gaucher cell is a large rounded or polyhedral cell varying in diameter from 20 to 80 µm. There is usually a single small, eccentric, deeply stained nucleus, but many cells have more than one nucleus. The cytoplasm appears palely eosinophilic with many wavy, thin fibrils giving it a wrinkled or striated appearance. The Gaucher cell is not vacuolated; the deposits of the cerebroside kerasin cannot be demonstrated with the usual fat stains but give a positive PAS reaction[385]. These cells accumulate in masses and sheets and often compress each other to produce bizarre shapes. The liver may be greatly enlarged and the biopsy appears macroscopically mottled and pale or uniformly grey.

In *Niemann-Pick's disease*[9, 139, 332] the Kupffer cells are enlarged because of their content of sphingomyelin. Three to fourfold increase in hepatic weight has been recorded, and both the liver and the biopsy are paler than normal. The cells are enlarged up to 90 µm in diameter, usually with a single, centrally placed nucleus and with a foamy vacuolated cytoplasm. In some cases these cells are scattered among the hepatocytes but in others the picture may be reversed, with scattered hepatocytes in areas dominated by Niemann-Pick cells. The content of sphingomyelin is preserved in H & E-stained sections but is best studied in frozen sections where it is positive with Sudan stains.

Polyvinyl pyrrolidone (PVP)[134, 135] known as a plasma expander and a stabilizer for Insipidin Retard may lead to the appearance in the Kupffer cells of globular homogeneous basophilic deposits thought to be macromolecules of PVP. The Kupffer cells are enlarged and occur singly or in small clusters (Fig. 125). Most often the nucleus is displaced toward the periphery of the cell.

In toxoplasmosis calcium deposists and rarely the organisms may be demonstrated[383], and in hepatic leishmaniasis Leishmania donovani may be found[85].

Morphological diagnosis: In the diagnosis of storage diseases, a careful appraisal of the cytoplasm of the Kupffer cells is important. H & E is the most important staining method but in cases with only slight changes appropriate special stains may be helpful. Immunofluorescent techniques are helpful for the identification of intracellular toxoplasma.

Differential diagnosis: The Niemann-Pick cells are foamy and stain with Sudan stains in frozen sections. They are, in contrast to the Gaucher cells, only slightly positive with PAS[9]. The Gaucher cells are wrinkled, without a foamy appearance, and do not stain with the Sudan dyes[133]. PVP is homogeneous, slightly basophilic and negative with PAS and Sudan stains[135].

Additional morphological findings: In Gaucher's disease fibrosis surrounding Gaucher cells, either lying singly or in clusters, may be seen. In some cases confluent fibrosis or bridging fibrosis occurs in connections with large groups of Gaucher cells[332]. In Niemann-Pick's disease the deposits of sphingomyelin in Kupffer cells are often accompanied by parenchymal changes, with bile stasis and giant cell formation[9]. Periportal fibrosis may occur.

Deposits of PVP are occasionally associated with a minor degree of focal necrosis and a mild inflammatory reaction but there is no fibrosis. Deposits of PVP are found in addition in reticuloendothelial cells in other organs, such as lymphnodes, bone marrow and spleen[134, 135].

Occurrence and significance: The inborn errors of lipid metabolism known as Gaucher's and Niemann-Pick's disease have been described in three and five different forms, respectively[332, 385]. Most of them involve the liver, but other organs with reticuloendothelial elements are also affected. These lesions are seldom seen in biopsy material and almost exclusively in biopsies from infants. The deposits of PVP in Kupffer cells are rare, and have scarcely any clinical significance[135].

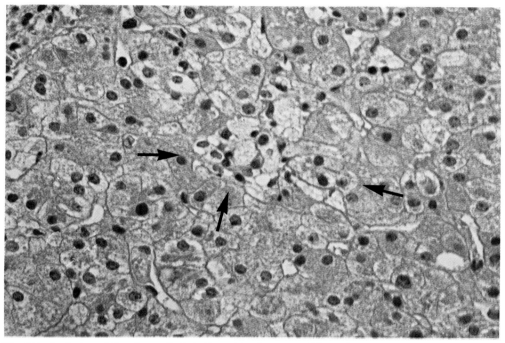

Fig. 124: A cluster of Gaucher cells is indicated in the center. The cells are large, slightly polyhedral with eccentric nuclei and with a rich, palely stained cytoplasm containing thin wavy fibrils (Needle biopsy, H & E x 270).

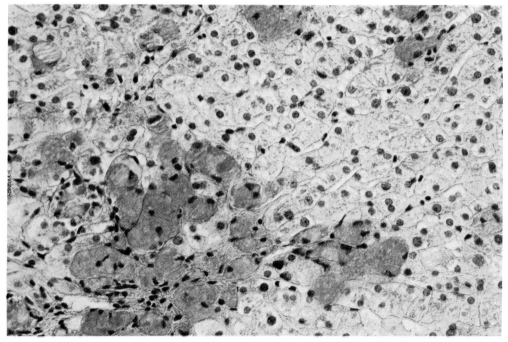

Fig. 125: Liver parenchyma from a patient with diabetes insipidus treated for decades with Insipidin Retard. The Kupffer cells are enlarged with large amounts of homogeneous dark colored cytoplasm (Needle biopsy, H & E x 270).

Hemopoiesis

Morphology: When hemopoietic tissue is present one finds smaller or larger foci in the sinusoids, often marginal in location. Ultrastructural investigations have made it probable that the hemopoietic foci are located in the space of Disse which is increased in width[108, 370, 394].

In the newborn and in infants remnants of hemopoietic tissue are often present. The foci are usually small and the picture is dominated by erythroblasts with relatively few white blood cell precursors. Megakaryocytes are absent or very scanty[108].

If present in older children and adults elements of all three cell series are usually found[394]. The distribution of the different cell types varies and frequently one may find foci of erythroblasts in between areas dominated by megakaryocytes. The megakaryocytes, which are the most readily recognizable of the various hemopoietic elements, are often more or less deformed compared to bone marrow megakaryocytes, probably because of adaptation to their sourroundings.

Morphological diagnosis: When hemopoiesis is widespread and comprises many megakaryocytes, the diagnosis is easy in H & E-stained sections and can usually be made at low magnification (Fig. 126 & 127). In cases with less pronounced changes and only small foci of erythropoiesis and myelopoiesis, Giemsa staining may be of help, but in our experience a systematic examination of serial sections always reveals a few megakaryocytes. The megakaryocytes represent the safest diagnostic criterion.

Differential diagnosis: Cellular infiltrates comprising erythropoiesis and myelopoiesis without megakaryocytes may present differential diagnostic problems against sinusoidal lining cell prominence and proliferation as well as against leukemic infiltrations[4] and malignant lymphomas[145, 215].

Hemopoietic tissue gives a more varied picture, with different cell types, than, do lining cell prominence and proliferation, and in the latter change many cells usually contain significant amounts of ceroid pigment.

Hemopoietic foci may occur together with leukemic infiltrates[4] or malignant lymphomas[215]. The latter are best recognized by the denser and more extensive cellular infiltrates with less variation in cell type but with morphological signs of malignancy. These include variation in form, size and stainability of the nuclei.

Additional morphological findings: It is not uncommon to see hemopoiesis as the only pathological finding in a liver biopsy. In some cases there may in addition be other changes such as non-specific inflammation or slight steatosis and, mainly when hemolysis is present one may find iron positive pigment, first in Kupffer cells and later in liver cells.

Occurrence and significance: Small foci of hemopoiesis occur normally in the liver of the newborn but they soon disappear. The finding later in life is consequently pathological. It must, however, be emphasized that a single or very few erythroblasts or even a megakaryocyte may be found in patients apparently without hematological disease[4].

Hemopoiesis in the liver is part of an extramedullary hemopoiesis, and the cause or causes of this condition are to be found either in the bone marrow (which can be either replaced or aplastic) or in a need for new formation of hemopoietic elements which cannot be met by the bone marrow. Hemopoiesis of the liver is most often seen in myelofibrosis but is also sometimes due to extensive bone marrow metastases, various aplastic conditions and severe forms of hemolytic anemia, megaloblastic anemia and leucocytosis[4].

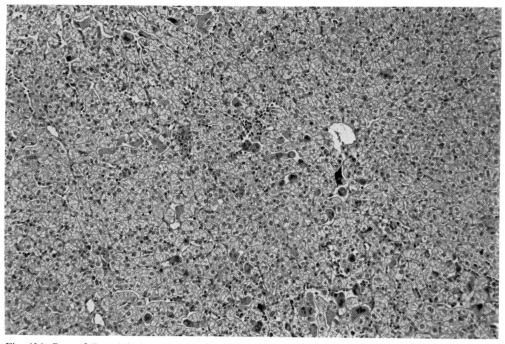

Fig. 126: Part of liver lobule with small portal tracts in the lower left corner and a central vein a little right of and above the middle. There are many cellular infiltrates comprising both small and very large cells in the sinusoids (Surgical biopsy, H & E x 110).

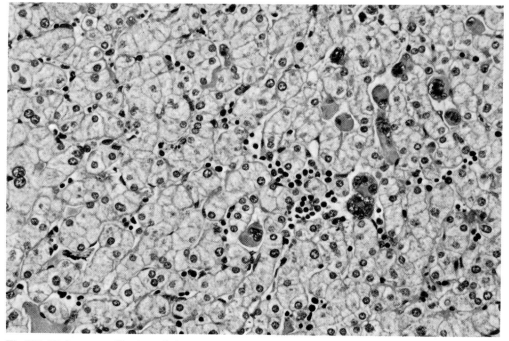

Fig. 127: Higher magnification of the same area as Fig. 126. Many megakaryocytes and other blood forming elements, in particular erythroblasts, are present in the sinusoids. From a patient with myelofibrosis (Surgical biopsy, H & E x 270).

Leukemic infiltrations

Morphology: The liver parenchyma, space of Disse and sinusoids may be affected in all forms of advanced leukemia[4, 186].

In acute lymphoblastic and acute myeloblastic leukemia the infiltration is massive, dense and diffuse (Fig. 128), with immature cells showing variation in form and size. The nuclei are large and often contain several nucleoli, and mitoses are common. A few megakaryocytes are usually demonstrable. The infiltration is virtually always continuous with similar infiltration in the portal tracts[4, 186].

In chronic myeloid leukemia the cellular infiltration is also diffusely distributed in the sinusoids[4, 329]. The infiltrates are nearly always more loosely structured than in acute leukemia (Fig. 129), and the cellular picture is more varied with varying proportions of promyelocytes, myelocytes and metamyelocytes. As in acute leukemia one can virtually always find continuity between parenchymal and portal infiltrates.

As previously pointed out (p. 62) the characteristic infiltrates in chronic lymphatic leukemia are mainly situated in the portal tracts[186]. They may, however, encroach on the parenchyma, and in some cases one may find infiltrates confined to the parenchyma. The parenchymal infiltrates consist of mature lymphocytic elements and they are more focal and better demarcated than other leukemic infiltrates.

In the rarer forms of leukemia such as erythroleukemia and monocytic leukemia the distribution of the cellular infiltrates is usually as in acute leukemia.

Morphological diagnosis: The identification of leukemic infiltrations is nearly always easy in H & E-stained sections, but a systematic examination of multiple sections is necessary for the recognition of the smallest foci.

Giemsa-stained sections may be of help for classification of the leukemia, but differentiation is especially difficult between acute lymphoblastic and acute myeloblastic forms, and a detailed diagnosis should only be made after comparison with a bone marrow aspirate.

Differential diagnosis: Acute leukemic infiltration may closely resemble the sinusoidal changes in infectious mononucleosis. In leukemia the infiltrates tend, however, to be more dense and the cells have larger and more pleomorphic nuclei, more nucleoli and more mitoses.

The infiltrates in chronic myeloid leukemia may have similarities with hemopoiesis[329, 374]. The leukemic infiltrates comprise different stages of myelopoiesis and as a rule no megakaryocytes or erythroblasts.

The infiltrates found in chronic lymphatic leukemia cannot be distinguished from the infiltrates which may arise in the course of a malignant lymphoma of lymphocytic type.

Additional morphological findings: There are no characteristic additional findings in the liver in leukemia. In anemia, steatosis may develop, in hemolytic conditions siderosis, and in pyemia focal liver cell necrosis with neutrophils. Not uncommonly foci of hemopoiesis may be seen in addition to leukemic infiltration[329].

Occurrence and significance: Leukemic infiltration of the liver js frequent in all forms of leukemia and nearly constant in the end stages[186]. The infiltrates can disappear completely during remission of the disease.

The demonstration of leukemic infiltration in a liver biopsy is only rarely of diagnostic importance but gives information on the extent of the disease[4, 329].

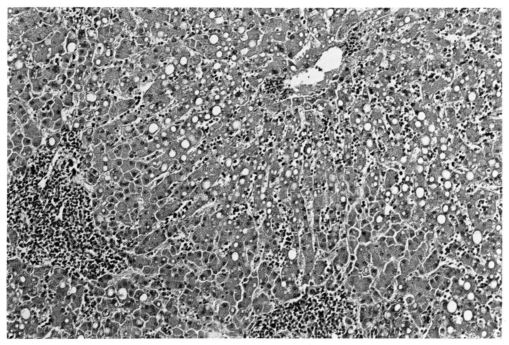

Fig. 128: Part of a liver lobule with a central vein (upper right) and two portal tracts. Dense infiltrates are present in the portal tracts and more diffuse infiltrates are seen in the sinusoids. From a patient with acute lymphoblastic leukemia (Needle biopsy, H & E x 110).

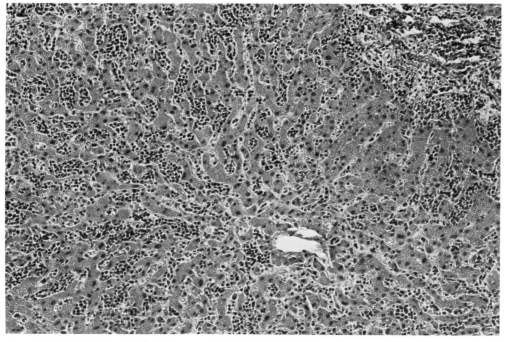

Fig. 129: Part of a liver lobule with a portal tract in the upper right corner and a central vein in the lower part of the middle third. A cellular infiltrate predominantly in the sinusoids is seen. From a patient with chronic myeloid leukemia (Needle biopsy, H & E x 110).

Metastases and malignant lymphoma

Morphology: Metastases may be of all sizes and are usually seen in the form of rounded nodules. They are to be found in both portal tracts and parenchyma[136]. All histological types occur but adenocarcinoma from the gastrointestinal tract and the breast and anaplastic carcinoma from the lung account for a large proportion[136]. Necrosis of the tumor tissue and varying degrees of inflammation are common[185]. In some cases, especially in metastases from small cell anaplastic bronchogenic carcinoma, the tumor cells may infiltrate along the space of Disse (Fig. 130) and thus give a characteristic picture with accentuation of the architecture of the liver cell plates.

All forms of malignant lymphoma may infiltrate the sinusoids and in most cases the portal tracts are also involved. In diffuse lymphoma of lymphocytic type the cells are closely set and vary only slightly in size, form and stainability[376]. The infiltrates are mainly found in the portal tracts and are most often well delineated, but they may extend into the parenchyma, and cases with pure parenchymal infiltrates occur.

In patients with diffuse lymphoma of histiocytic type the infiltrates in the liver are less well demarcated and more often both portal tracts and parenchyma are involved[377].

Only a minority of patients with lymphoma of Hodgkins' type show infiltrates in the liver[215]. When present, one or more infiltrates of varying size and shape are found involving portal tracts and/or parenchyma (Fig. 131). Reed-Sternberg cells are often sparse[16].

For primary tumors of the liver see chapter III.

Morphological diagnosis: H & E is suitable for the demonstration of secondary malignant tumors in the liver parenchyma. The diagnosis is usually easy since relatively large deposits are usually present at the same time in one or more portal tracts. Small isolated parenchymal infiltrates may, however, be overlooked unless multiple sections are examined.

In some cases of malignant lymphoma with only slight infiltration of the liver it is only possible to give a presumptive diagnosis. Multiple sections are often valuable, especially for the demonstration of Reed-Sternberg cells.

Differential diagnosis: Metastatic carcinoma seldom presents problems with regard to malignancy but only in the minority of cases does the histological appearance of the tumor clearly indicate the site of primary growth. Some cases of small cell anaplastic bronchogenic carcinoma may give a false impression of malignant lymphoma, but the cell nuclei are darker and the variation in size is greater.

Malignant lymphomas usually cause no differential diagnostic problems as most are accompanied by characteristic portal changes.

Additional morphological findings: The parenchyma often shows cholestasis and other features of bile duct obstruction. Localized histological features of obstruction in patients without jaundice is suggestive of metastasis. In malignant lymphoma the additional changes in the liver parenchyma are usually minimal and non-specific.

Occurrence and significance: Malignant tumor tissue is common in most biopsy series, and it is fairly common for the diagnosis of malignant disease to be made first by liver biopsy. It may, however, be impossible to identify the primary site and sometimes, especially in poorly differentiated tumors, it may be impossible to differentiate between primary and secondary carcinomas (p. 194).

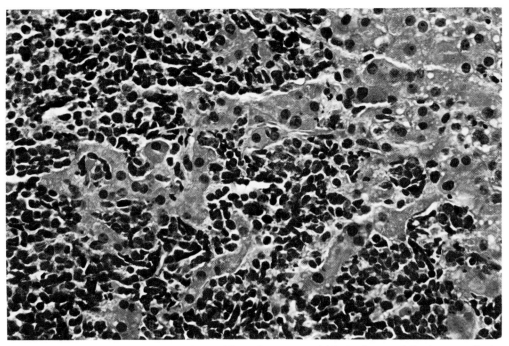

Fig. 130: Tumor cells in liver parenchyma. There is an appreciable tendency of the tumor cells to spread along the sinusoids. From a patient with anaplastic bronchogenic carcinoma (Needle biopsy, H & E x 270).

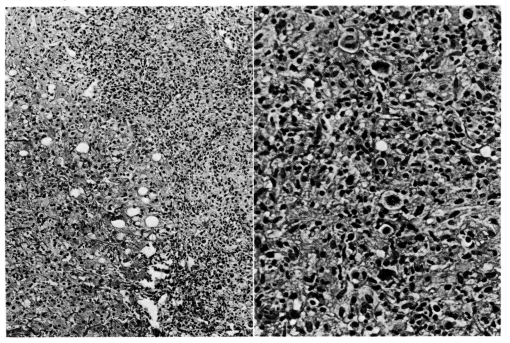

Fig. 131: Left. Small magnification of a Hodgkin infiltrate in the liver. The border towards uninvolved parenchyma is irregular (x 110). Right. Higher magnification of the infiltrate showing scattered Reed-Sternberg cells (Autopsy, H & E x 270).

Amyloid

Morphology: Parenchymal amyloid is found in the space of Disse between the walls of the sinusoids and the adjacent hepatic cells, closely applied to the Kupffer cells[357].

The material is homogeneous and pink on H & E (Fig. 132). It may affect all parts of the lobule and in most cases all zones are equally involved. A mid-zonal and periportal over-weight is sometimes found. When deposition is massive the liver cells undergo atrophy and the sinusoids are narrowed. The amount of parenchymal amyloid may vary from lobule to lobule and from biopsy to biopsy in the same patient[75].

Electron microscopical investigations have shown the same fine structure as in amyloid elsewhere[74, 75, 222]. Fine fibrils distend the space of Disse, and are closely related to Kupffer as well as to parenchymal cells.

The gross appearance is in well-developed cases a firm and waxy enlarged liver with normal form but with rounded borders[75].

Morphological diagnosis: Whereas the amyloid is easily seen in routine stains when larger amounts are present, it is easily overlooked when sparse. The identification of amyloid needs special stains[75]. Its chemical nature is not completely known and may vary from case to case. Amyloid is PAS-positive and stains red with Congo red. It is stained metachromatically, especially in secondary amyloidosis, with methyl- and crystal violet (Fig. 133). In polarized light a strong green birefringence is seen after staining with Congo red and silver birefringence after thioflavin[238]. The latter is generally believed to be the most reliable method for demonstration of amyloid light microscopically. Ultrastructurally amyloid has a characteristic fibrillar structure[222].

Amyloid may also be demonstrated by fluorescent microscopy. Parenchymal amyloidosis is very diffusely distributed in the liver and sampling error is negligible.

Differential diagnosis: Because of its amorphous appearance, amyloid should offer no difficulties in diagnosis, but as mentioned above it may be overlooked when there are only small amounts.

Additional morphological findings: Amyloid is often found in otherwise normal liver tissue. In some cases amyloid deposits may also be seen in portal tracts, localized in the walls of hepatic artery or portal venous branches[357] (p. 60). Involvement of central veins is rare and may in exceptional cases give rise to venous outflow obstruction.

Intrahepatic cholestasis is uncommon but may be present in both primary and secondary amyloidosis.

Occurrence and significance: Parenchymal amyloid is seen in more than 80 per cent of patients with secondary amyloidosis[27] and in more than half of patients with primary amyloidosis[366].

Secondary (perireticular) amyloidosis may follow chronic disorders such as rheumatoid arthritis, tuberculosis, suppurative long-lasting osteomyelitis, ulcerative colitis, Crohn's disease, leprosy and Hodgkins' disease and in addition to the liver the kidneys and spleen are most often affected[75].

Primary (pericollagen) amyloidosis is rare and without preexisting disease[366]. The liver is only rarely involved and the amyloid is found mainly in tongue, heart, skin, muscles and lungs.

The progression of the hepatic amyloid is unpredictable. Serial biopsies have shown apparently stable amyloidosis in some cases and rapid progression in others[202].

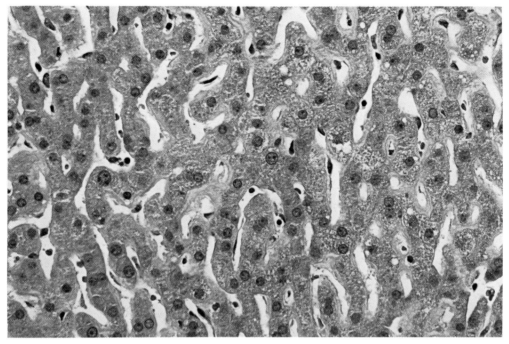

Fig. 132: Liver cell plates and sinusoids from a biopsy with preserved lobular architecture. In some areas an eosinophilic thickening of the sinusoidal walls can be noticed. From a patient with secondary amyloidosis (Needle biopsy, H & E x 270).

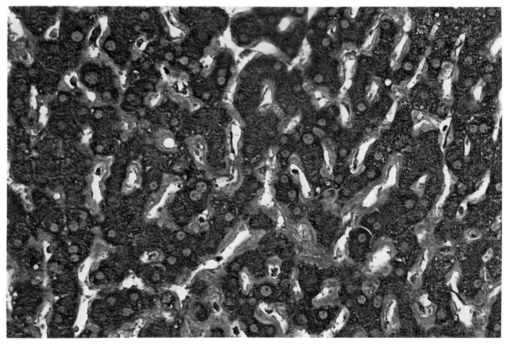

Fig. 133: Part of the same lobule as above. Serial section stained with methyl violet. The metachromatic (red) material, the amyloid, is seen with greater ease and in much larger amounts than in H & E (Needle biopsy, methyl violet x 270).

Normal

Morphology: The central vein is regarded as the center of the conventional lobule, and virtually all sinusoids empty into these smallest roots of the hepatic venous system[122] (Fig. 134 & 135). Only in few areas do sinusoids connect directly with larger veins. Central veins enter almost perpendicularly into sublobular veins. The sublobular veins converge to form collecting veins which ultimately unite to form the main hepatic veins. Most commonly there are three main veins, two draining the right lobe and one draining the left. The number and size of the hepatic veins are, however, quite variable.

In the Rappaport acinus[301] which is centered around an axis comprising terminal portal venules, hepatic arterioles and bile ducts, the central veins are peripherally located ("terminal hepatic veins") (p. 22, Fig. 11).

A little connective tissue, especially in older persons, surrounds the central and especially the sublobular veins. It is seen as a fine mantle of collagen fibers (Fig. 139).

In most biopsies the lumen is empty but sometimes varying number of erythrocytes are present. The lumen is lined by endothelial cells and sometimes also by Kupffer cells.

It is exceptional when veins larger than sublobular veins are represented in needle biopsies.

Morphological diagnosis: The histological recognition of normal central veins is usually easy. Low magnification should be used, and sections stained for reticulin and collagen fibers as well as with H & E. The differentiation between tangentially cut central veins and sublobular veins is made by the size of the lumen and the amount of connective tissue in the wall.

Differential diagnosis: The most important differential diagnostic problem has to do with the parenchymal nodules in macronodular cirrhosis since parts of these may show one-cell-thick plates with a certain degree of radial arrangement. The irregular distribution of the efferent vessels helps to exclude normal central veins. The lack of normal appearing connective tissue mantles in the walls is also important.

Additional morphological findings: Liver tissue with preserved and normal central veins may be completely normal but most of the parenchymal and portal changes described in this atlas may be found in livers with preserved central veins.

Occurrence and significance: In most series the majority of biopsies show preserved central veins. One of the most important considerations in liver biopsy diagnosis is the exclusion of cirrhosis. If, in the interpretation of a biopsy, one finds portal tracts and central veins regularly spaced throughout the whole biopsy with an intervening distance of about 400 to 700 μm, and in addition a radial arrangement of liver cells around the central veins is observed, then the normal architecture is preserved.

There are in the normal liver no direct anastomoses between on the one side hepatic artery and portal vein radicles and on the other side ramifications of the hepatic vein[174, 227]. The blood must pass through the sinusoids. The liver works under normal conditions as a kind of filter, and the hepatic venous blood is nearly always sterile. Also antigens are filtered in large amounts[223].

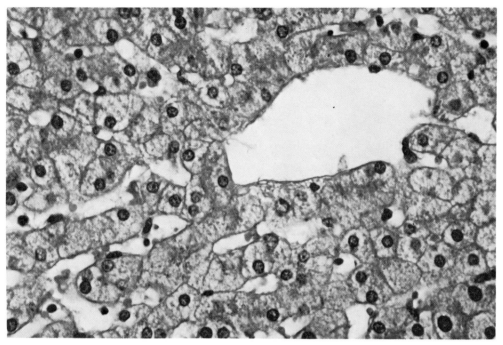

Fig. 134: Normal central vein with adjacent part of the parenchyma. Two openings of sinusoids into the lumen of the vein are seen in the right side of the wall (Needle biopsy, H & E x 270).

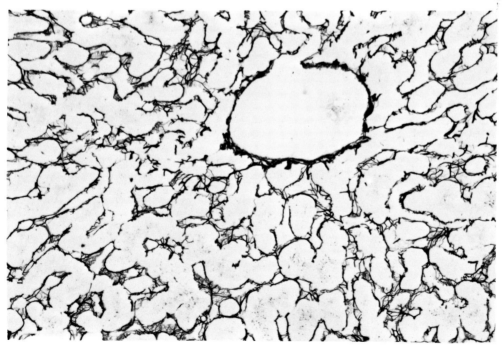

Fig. 135: Another section of the same area with the same central vein shows the condensed reticulin fibers in the wall. A van Gieson-stained section of the same vein disclosed quite a few small bundles of collagen fibers (Needle biopsy, reticulin x 270).

Occlusion

Morphology: Occlusion of hepatic vein radicles are very rare and are most often seen in connection with *Budd Chiari's syndrome* and *veno-occlusive disease*[304].

Recent thrombosis of the smallest veins, central and sublobular veins is seen in some cases of the Budd Chiari syndrome and is secondary to occlusion of the inferior vena cava or the hepatic veins and their tributaries[86, 159, 304]. The congestion may be so abrupt and severe as to produce necrosis of most of the hepatocytes, and in these cases most of the lobule is replaced by blood with only a rim of normal appearing liver cells at the periphery. In other cases, when the onset is more gradual, the central area with blood and fibrin is surrounded by a zone of liver tissue with dilated and usually empty sinusoids but with a characteristic infiltration of erythrocytes into the space of Disse[199] (Fig. 136). In later stages the thrombi organize (Fig. 137) to a collagenous core from which collagen strands may extend in an arachnoid fashion into the surrounding collapsed parenchyma.

Veno-occlusive disease is characterized by occlusion of the central and sublobular veins, whereas the larger veins are not affected[42]. The obstruction consists of a newly-formed subendothelial loose connective tissue, and in the early stages there is also often centrilobular sinusoidal dilatation and confluent necrosis. Later mainly centrilobular fibrosis and eventually cirrhosis may develop.

Morphological diagnosis: In early veno-occlusive disease the obliteration of the small vein radicles is characteristic but in the later stage the veins are often difficult to demonstrate in the fibrous tissue, but stains for collagen may be helpful in outlining the veins.

Differential diagnosis: In confluent centrilobular necrosis provoked by cardiac shock[52, 73], sinusoidal dilatation of the adjacent parenchyma may be conspicuous, and the necrosis is usually associated with hemorrhage, but venous occlusion is not a prominent feature.

The picture in Budd Chiari's syndrome is often indistinguishable from those of any obstruction of the hepatic venous flow such as right-sided heart failure.

Additional morphological findings: It is characteristic that the portal tracts for a long time remain normal or show only slight, non-specific inflammatory reaction.

Occurrence and significance: As indicated above occlusion of the hepatic vein and/or its radicles is rare. The occlusion in Budd Chiari's syndrome may be due either to a web[159] (congenital in the vena cava) or to a mass[255] (e.g. thrombus, tumor) in the main veins or in the hepatic vein radicles. Passive congestion, especially with extravasation of erythrocytes, in the absence of heart failure suggests the disease[199]. Common causes for thrombosis are myeloproliferative syndrome[304], oral contraceptives[355], radiation hepatitis[304], tumors[230] (liver, adrenal, kidney), graft versus host reaction and paroxysmal nocturnal hemoglobinuria[255].

Most cases of veno-occlusive disease have been found in Jamaica in young children with a history of exposure to pyrrolozidine alkaloids from crytalaria and senecio plants[42]. Both Budd Chiari's syndrome and veno-occlusive disease may be seen in acute, subacute and chronic forms.

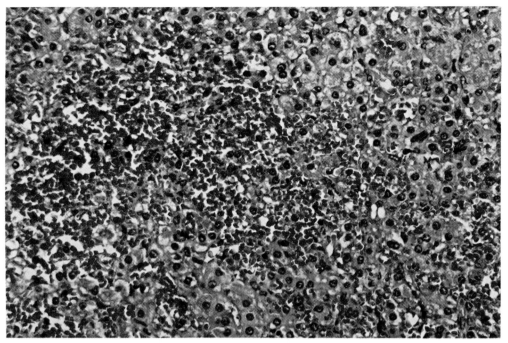

Fig. 136: Widespread and pronounced extravasation of erythrocytes in liver parenchyma in association with extended confluent necrosis. From a patient with Budd Chiari's syndrome (Surgical biopsy, H & E x 110).

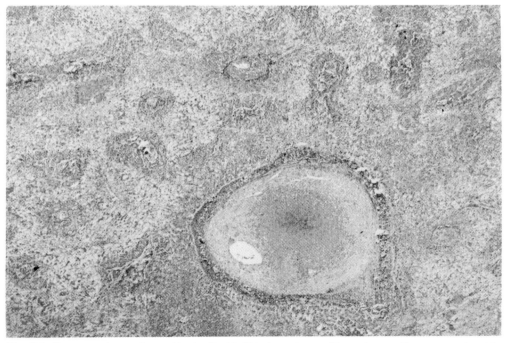

Fig. 137: From another patient with the Budd Chiari syndrome. Extensive confluent necrosis with only a small rim of preserved liver cells around portal tracts and a partly organized thrombus in a large vein are seen (Autopsy, van Gieson x 30).

Normal

Morphology: Biochemical research has in recent years demonstrated the existence of at least 8 different types of collagen molecules[235, 274]. Of these type I and type II are the best defined. The exact composition of type III and type IV is still hardly quite elucidated, while knowledge of the remaining collagen types is at the moment scanty. So far types I, III and IV have been identified in normal and cirrhotic liver.

A clear histologic distinction between the different types of collagen molecules cannot be made at the moment. In all probability the different histological methods such as van Gieson's picrofuchsin, variants of Mallory's phosphomolybdic or phosphotungstic acid aniline blue method, and silver impregnation following oxidation show up all biochemical types of collagen, but possibly with varying intensity.

The fibers in the normal connective tissue of the liver capsule, portal tracts and around many hepatic vein radicles stain red with the van Gieson stain as we perform it (see technical appendix). In this atlas fibers which are stained in this manner are called *collagen fibers* and these chiefly represent collagen type I. Fibrosis denotes increased amounts of collagen fibers.

The silver impregnation methods chiefly show up what histologically has been designated *reticulin fibers,* and this is the term we have used in this atlas. The biochemical equivalent of reticulin cannot at the moment be determined but probably represents both collagen type III and type IV as well as possibly other as yet undetermined types.

The liver has a fibrous tissue capsule which invests the vessels and the hepatic ducts as they enter the liver. It continues to support the portal tracts as they branch so that even the smallest branches lie in a mantle of collagenous tissue.

The capsular connective tissue contains many thick bundles of collagen fibers (Fig. 138). The thickness of the capsule varies from person to person and in a substantial number of cases one can find in the subcapsular region 1–2 mm thick fibrous bundles extending from the capsule into the parenchyma, giving the latter an irregular architecture[266].

Like that of the capsule, the connective tissue of the portal tracts is dominated by collagen fibers, which in van Gieson-stained sections are seen to form short and thick bundles. The portal tracts contain in addition a network of reticulin fibers which form a concentric zone around vessels and bile ducts and which in the limiting membrane area are in direct continuity with the fibers of the reticulin of the parenchyma. Often a little connective tissue also surrounds the central and especially the sublobular veins, mainly in older persons. It is seen as a fine mantle of small thick bundles in stain for collagen fibers (Fig. 139).

The lobule is supported by fine reticulin fibers lying in the space of Disse, whereas collagen fibers are normally lacking in the parenchyma.

Differential diagnosis: Large portal tracts and portal tracts with ramifications may imitate fibrosis. Enlarged portal tracts with inflammatory processes with edema and many inflammatory cells may, similarly, give the impression of fibrosis, especially if stain for collagen fibers is not applied.

Additional morphological findings: Biopsies without fibrosis are found not only in normal liver tissue but also in many commonly occurring conditions such as acute hepatitis, nonspecific reactive hepatitis, steatosis and the majority of drug lesions. In chronic persistent hepatitis there is only minimal or no fibrosis[89, 380].

Occurrence and significance: Most series of biopsies thus include a large number of biopsies without fibrosis. Absence of fibrosis is of essential diagnostic significance since it helps to exclude, for example chronic aggressive hepatitis[89] and cirrhosis[7, 380] with a high degree of probability.

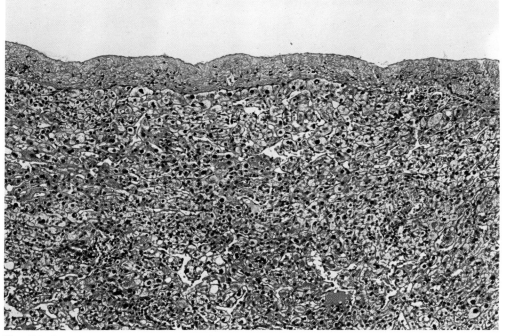

Fig. 138: Capsular and subcapsular area of a surgical biopsy without pathological changes. Note the thickness of the capsule and the dense structure of its connective tissue (Surgical biopsy, H & E x 30).

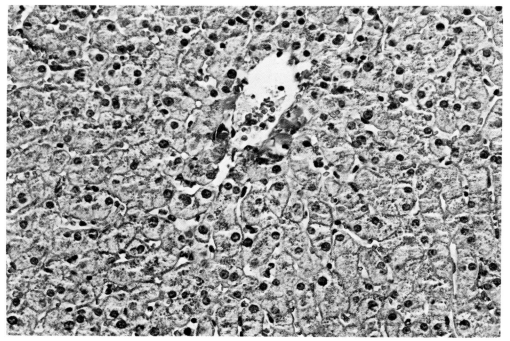

Fig. 139: Central vein area from a normal liver. There are relatively thick and collagen rich connective tissue bundles in parts of the vein wall. Many of the liver cells contain lipofuscin granules (Needle biopsy, van Gieson x 270).

Portal fibrosis

Morphology: Fibrosis in the portal tracts may be found in pure forms but is usually associated with periportal fibrosis. A portal fibrosis may be well demarcated and without special localization as it is seen in the healing or healed stages of granulomatous diseases such as sarcoidosis or miliary tuberculosis[131, 190].

Another form of portal fibrosis is an increase of connective tissue around bile ducts, so-called periductal fibrosis[373] (Fig. 140). The lesion is usually concentric around the duct and with onion-skin appearance possibly with areas with hyalinization. In some cases the centrally located bile duct may be inconspicuous or even missing in some sections (Fig. 141).

In hepatoportal sclerosis there is thickening of the intima of the larger portal vein branches, sometimes with recanalized thrombosis, whereas the smaller branches usually look normal. In old cases scarified areas without significant portal vein branches may be found[233, 315].

In all three forms of portal fibrosis slight to moderate inflammation mainly with lymphocytes and histiocytes may be found but it is not the rule.

A special type is congenital hepatic fibrosis[163, 183] (p. 52).

Morphological diagnosis: Prerequisites for an accurate diagnosis are large biopsies with several portal tracts and serial sections. The changes in hepatoportal sclerosis can as a rule only be demonstrated in surgical biopsies since only few needle biopsies comprise the large portal vein branches affected in this condition.

Differential diagnosis: In some cases it may be difficult or even impossible to distinguish portal from periportal fibrosis. Only by use of serial sections may an accurate diagnosis be given.

Additional morphological findings: Portal fibrosis may occur as the only change but is often accompanied by for instance changes in centrally located bile ducts or granulomatous lesions.

Occurrence and significance: Focal accumulation of fibrous tissue in the portal tracts is seen in many conditions and is usually not associated with portal hypertension.

Periductal fibrosis is a common findings in long-lasting extrahepatic biliary obstruction[327e] but may also be found in intrahepatic lesions such as primary biliary cirrhosis[153].

So-called sclerosing cholangitis is a lesion of the extrahepatic bile ducts characterized by a chronic portal inflammation and gradually increasing periductal fibrosis[340]. Sclerosing cholangitis is found in some patients with severe and longstanding ulcerative colitis but may also occur in patients with Crohn's disease and in cases with orbital and retroperitoneal fibrosis.

Hepatoportal sclerosis is an ill-defined disease both clinically, morphologically and pathogenetically. In the literature a variety of terms are used, such as obliterative portal venopathy, hepatolienal fibrosis or Banti's syndrome[275]. These terms imply a disorder, different from cirrhosis, in which splenic enlargement is associated with presinusoidal portal hypertension and varying degrees of portal fibrosis. The same combination of portal fibrosis with portal hypertension and splenomegaly has been observed in patients treated with arsenic[244] and other noxious agents and in workers exposed to vinyl chloride[284].

Portal fibrosis may also be found in schistosomiasis. In severe cases scarring around the portal vein tributaries and possibly granulomas are seen[391].

In some instances fibrosis is found as the only change in a biopsy, i.e. without for instance signs of hepatitis, steatosis or cirrhosis. In such cases the main diagnosis is portal fibrosis. A similar descriptive diagnosis may be valid for the other types of fibrosis.

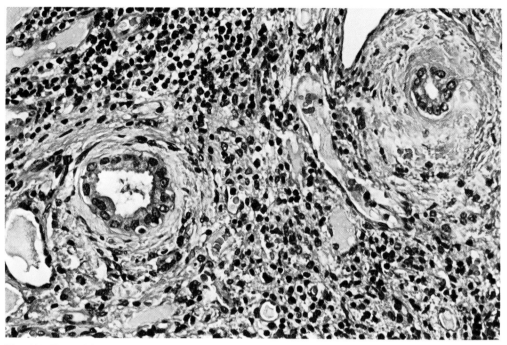

Fig. 140: Part of large portal tract with two bile ducts. Both are surrounded by increased amounts of connective tissue. Around the left duct onion-skin appearance is seen, whereas hyalinization is conspicuous around the right (Surgical biopsy, H & E x 270).

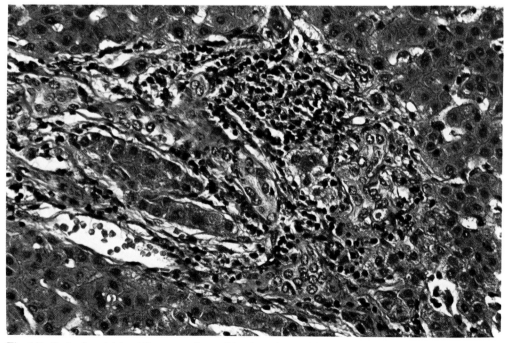

Fig. 141: Part of portal tract from a patient with ulcerative colitis and sclerosing cholangitis. There is periductular and partly diffuse fibrosis which contains lymphocytes and suppressed bile ducts (Needle biopsy, H & E x 270).

Focal fibrosis

Morphology: In liver tissue with preserved lobular architecture one may in the parenchyma find not only periportal, centrilobular and bridging fibrosis (described on the following pages), but also new connective tissue irregularly distributed in the lobules. *Focal fibrosis* and *pericellular fibrosis* can often be distinguished although transitional forms occur.

Focal fibrosis is seen as rounded or partly stellate areas of newly formed collagen fibers. As a rule they fill small or relatively small defects of the liver cell plates and are, in the early stages, associated with Kupffer cell proliferation and infiltration by lymphocytes and plasma cells and sometimes with granulomas.

Focal fibrosis is especially common after lipogranulomas[57] and alcoholic hepatitis[56] and is also a frequent finding in healing granulomatous diseases such as sarcoidosis (Fig. 142)[190]. The number and size of the lesions depend on the severity of the original disease and its dissemination in the liver tissue.

Focal fibrosis following lipogranulomas[57] or epithelioid cell granulomas[190] are without characteristic zonal distribution, whereas the lesions following alcoholic hepatitis mainly are centrilobular[56].

Morphological diagnosis: Multiple sections stained for collagen fibers are necessary for the diagnosis of focal fibrosis and for the exact evaluation of the number and extent of the lesions (Fig. 143).

Differential diagnosis: When examination is restricted to H & E-stained sections and sections stained for reticulin fibers, focal necrosis or granulomatous structures may be misinterpreted as fibrosis.

Additional morphological findings: If the etiological factor is still active, one may find changes such as alcoholic hepatitis, lipogranulomas or other forms of granulomas.

Occurrence and significance: Focal fibrosis is most commonly seen in liver biopsies from alcoholics with steatosis together with alcoholic hepatitis[66]. Focal fibrosis is usually reversible, but it is probable that larger lesions may sometimes be precursors of portal-central bridging fibrosis since it is sometimes possible to demonstrate intermediate stages apparently representing transitions between confluent focal fibrosis and true portal-central septa[66].

The small focal fibrotic lesions arising after lipogranulomas are most often reversible[57] and the same holds true for the usually somewhat larger lesions arising after sarcoidosis.

Many and more or less confluent granulomas in sarcoidosis may sometimes, however, give rise to development of portal-central bridging fibrosis which again may be a preliminary to the development of a cirrhosis[216]

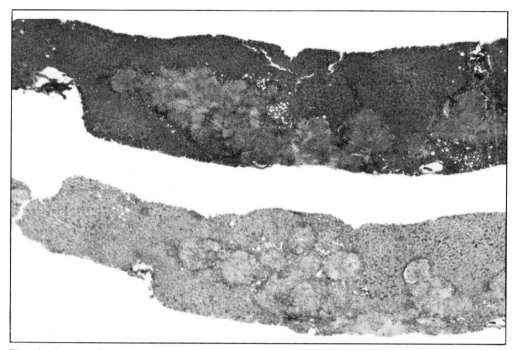

Fig. 142: Survey of needle biopsy with a large amount of mainly healed, fibrotic granulomas in both portal tracts and parenchyma. Sarcoidosis. Compare H & E (upper) and van Gieson (lower specimen) (Needle biopsy, H & E and van Gieson x 30).

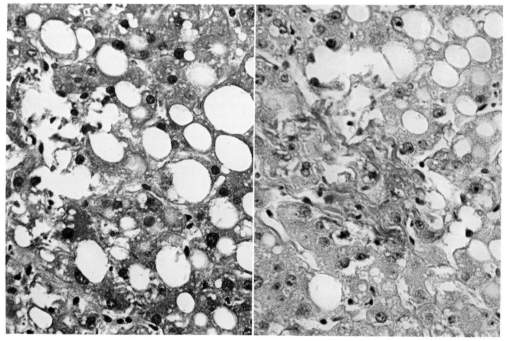

Fig. 143: Focal fibrosis probably following alcoholic hepatitis. Left. H & E-stained section shows steatosis whereas the fibrosis is inconspicuous. Right. Same area with van Gieson staining (Needle biopsy, x 270).

Pericellular fibrosis

Morphology: Whereas it is agreed that focal fibrosis arises after focal liver cell necrosis, there is no general agreement about the so-called pericellular fibrosis. It has been claimed that pericellular fibrosis may develop without or with only minimal preceding parenchymal necrosis[274]. Bundles of collagen are seen around single or small groups of non-necrotic but usually degenerated and especially enlarged hepatocytes often with empty looking cytoplasm. This form of fibrosis is usually, but not always, seen in the centrilobular part of the parenchyma and in relation to bridging fibrosis. A similar form of fibrosis is sometimes seen around histiocytes containing excess stored material, in particular iron[182].

The pericellular fibrosis may vary from cases with collagen surrounding a single cell or small groups of cells, to cases comprising substantial parts of lobules. In sections stained for collagen fibers a characteristic "chicken wire"-like picture is seen in small magnifications.

The development of collagen fibers is as a rule preceded by an increase in the amount of reticulin in the same area[182]. The pericellular fibrosis is nearly always accompanied by some infiltration by inflammatory cells in the early stages. The histiocytes may contain ceroid. Later the inflammation often subsides.

Morphological diagnosis: In order to recognize pericellular fibrosis with certainty sections stained for collagen fibers must be examined (Fig. 144 & 145). In the early phases one finds isolated liver cells or small groups surrounded by sparse loosely arranged, fine collagen fibers. There are often connections to neighboring central veins. Later the bundles of collagen become coarser and may eventually undergo hyalinization.

Differential diagnosis: Without the use of stain for collagen fibers pericellular fibrosis may be overlooked, just as areas of focal liver cell necrosis with collapse of the reticulin network but without true new fiber formation may be misinterpreted as pericellular fibrosis.

Pericellular fibrosis is sometimes seen in connection with both focal fibrosis and large fibrotic lesions such as bridging fibrosis.

Additional morphological findings: Pericellular fibrosis is most often found together with steatosis and alcoholic hepatitis, possibly in connection with centrilobular fibrosis, but it may also be seen in relation to piecemeal necrosis, mainly in chronic aggressive hepatitis.

Occurrence and significance: Investigation of follow-up biopsies has shown that pericellular fibrosis is reversible to a large extent. On the other hand it is probable that extended pericellular fibrosis may be restrictive to the nutrition of the liver cells, resulting in necrosis and thereby forming the basis for the development of larger fibrous septa, for instance of bridging fibrosis.

The pericellular fibrosis seen in chronic alcoholics is mainly centrilobular and is often combined with focal fibrosis following multiple, dispersed and small necrotic lesions as sometimes found in alcoholic hepatitis. In this way the centrilobular lattice network of collagen in alcoholics, known as central hyaline sclerosis, may be explained[113].

A similar "chicken-wire" picture may also be seen in severe cases of acute hepatitis and chronic hepatitis. The fibrosis is as a rule mainly periportal or diffusely distributed.

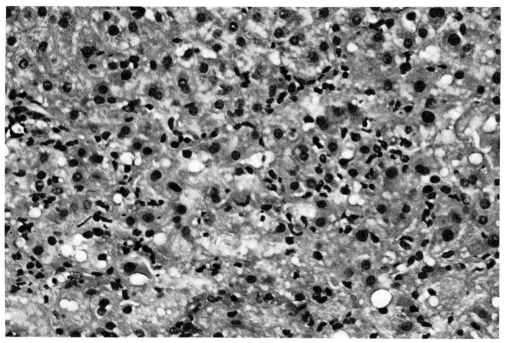

Fig. 144: Liver parenchyma from a patient with chronic alcoholism. A slight steatosis and some focal sinusoidal lining cell proliferation are recognizable (Needle biopsy, H & E x 270).

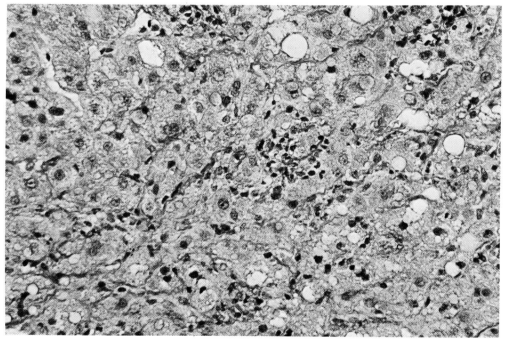

Fig. 145: Same areas as Fig. 144. Delicate collagen fibers are visible partly along the sinusoids, partly surrounding single liver cells or small groups of cells (pericellular fibrosis) (Needle biopsy, van Gieson x 270).

Periportal fibrosis

Morphology: Fibrosis involving smaller or larger areas of the parts of the lobules which are located around the portal tracts is called periportal fibrosis[31, 285] (Fig. 146). In the early phases one can, especially in van Gieson-stained sections, see a wide difference in the character of the newly formed connective tissue and the original, as the newly formed fibers are thinner and only have a very slight tendency to be arranged in bundles[94] (Fig. 147). The older the fibrosis becomes the more does the appearance become similar the original portal connective tissue. This process takes months, usually years[94]. Thus in a chronic aggressive hepatitis which has lasted for years one can usually still see a conspicuous difference between the newly formed and the original connective tissue. If the processes in the adjacent parenchyma remain active, liver cell necrosis and inflammation are present.

In many cases most typically seen in relation to the preterminal portal tracts, the periportal fibrosis comprises a zone which involves the whole or nearly the whole circumference of the tract, although this zone is usually of somewhat variable thickness. In other cases only a part of the circumference is fibrotic.

In still other cases longer or shorter connective tissue bands directed towards other portal tracts or towards central veins are seen mainly in relation to the smallest portal tracts. These bands or septa consist of collagen fibers and constitute bridging fibrosis, portal-portal bridging fibrosis when they connect portal tracts[31, 144], and portal-central bridging fibrosis when they connect portal tracts and central veins[31, 40, 143] (p. 162).

Morphological diagnosis: The precise recognition of periportal fibrosis can, as the other forms of fibrosis, only be made with certainty on sections stained for collagen fibers. It is a further prerequisite that the biopsy is large and comprises numerous lobules, and it is recommended to use many sections in order to exclude cirrhosis.

Differential diagnosis: With the use of H & E – and reticulin-stained sections only, that is to say without sections stained for collagen fibers, periportal liver cell necrosis may simulate periportal fibrosis, especially when necrosis is extensive and accompanied by substantial collapse of the reticulin framework.

Additional morphological findings: Periportal fibrosis is virtually always accompanied by bile duct proliferation and most often by inflammatory cells, and in the surrounding parenchyma liver cell necrosis and inflammation are common. A typical example is chronic aggressive hepatitis (p. 176). Another example is longstanding large duct obstruction (p. 186). If the histological activity has ceased, one can find mature connective tissue without or virtually without inflammation, where the parenchyma is free of liver cell necrosis.

Occurrence and significance: Periportal fibrosis is a prerequisite for the diagnosis of chronic aggressive hepatitis[89] and is also common in long-standing obstruction of the larger bile ducts[291]. If the fibrosis is extensive and in particular if there is conspicuous portal-central bridging fibrosis in addition to liver cell necrosis and inflammation, development of cirrhosis is very probable.

Periportal fibrosis can be reversible, as can many other forms of fibrosis. This is particularly so in younger persons with chronic aggressive hepatitis[58], and postoperatively in patients in whom obstruction to the larger bile ducts has been corrected[327c].

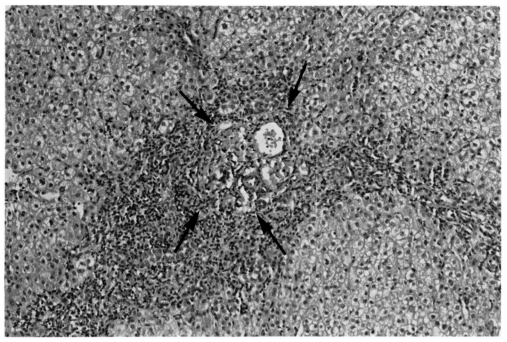

Fig. 146: Medium-sized portal tract with moderate to severe periportal fibrosis giving a stellate appearance. The original portal tract, indicated by arrows, can to some degree be recognized. Chronic aggressive hepatitis. (Needle biopsy, H & E x 110).

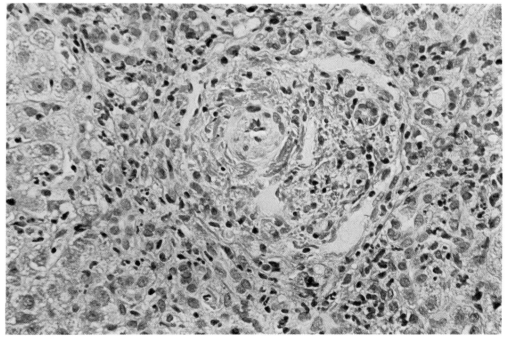

Fig. 147: Small portal tract with moderate periportal fibrosis with bile duct proliferation. There is a marked difference between the mature connective tissue of the original tract and the newly formed periportal fibrotic tissue (Needle biopsy, van Gieson x 270).

Centrilobular fibrosis

Morphology: Like periportal fibrosis, fibrosis in centrilobular areas can vary in extent, but is usually more or less in direct continuity with the wall of the central vein.

The newly formed connective tissue is formed as a consequence of centrilobular, so-called confluent liver cell necrosis, which is met with first and foremost in cardiogenic shock[73] (Fig. 148), in some forms of acute hepatitis[375], in exacerbation periods of chronic aggressive hepatitis[239], and in severe alcoholic hepatitis[281]. During the first few weeks after the development of the necrosis collapse of the reticulin network is seen, possibly with an increase in reticulin fibers. The fibrosis develops gradually, but it takes many months, most often several years, before the new connective tissue contains as many collagen fibers as the normal connective tissue of the liver.

The extent and outline of the fibrosis varies as indicated above. It may be seen as a poorly developed, irregular area around the central vein, but it is often characteristic, in particular when the fibrosis is substantial, that the fibrotic areas has an extent which corresponds closely to zone 3 of Rappaport's acinus[300]. Larger zones of fibrosis may connect central vein areas (central-central bridging fibrosis), or central vein areas and portal tracts (portal-central bridging fibrosis).

The connective tissue is often, particularly in alcoholics, without sharp delineation with extensions of varying size and shape stretching in between the neighboring liver cells (Fig. 149). In such cases the fibrous tissue is often more or less hyalinized ("central hyaline sclerosis")[113].

Morphological diagnosis: The diagnosis of centrilobular fibrosis can as a rule only be made satisfactorily in sections stained for collagen fibers. The liver tissue must have preserved lobular architecture, and only in well-orientated and processed biopsies and with the simultaneous use of serial sections is it possible to evaluate with reasonable certainly the extent of the fibrosis and the absence or presence of bridging fibrosis.

Differential diagnosis: Without the use of sections stained for collagen fibers, centrilobular necrosis may be mistaken for centrilobular fibrosis. Particularly in sections stained for reticulin fibers the collapse of these fibers may imitate fibrosis.

Additional morphological findings: In the parenchyma adjacent to the centrilobular fibrosis one may sometimes find necrosis, depending on the age and activity of the processes. Old fibrosis without activity is surrounded by liver cells without special characteristics.

If the processes are still active one may find, depending on the primary disease, such changes as dilatation of the sinusoids or features of acute hepatitis, chronic hepatitis or alcoholic hepatitis.

Occurrence and significance: Centrilobular fibrosis, sometimes with bridging fibrosis, is characteristically seen after severe attacks of cardiogenic shock[52], acute viral hepatitis[40] and alcoholic hepatitis[113], and after some drugs and toxins[187]. Centrilobular fibrosis without bridging fibrosis seen after acute virale hepatitis does not seem to predispose to cirrhosis[265] but in chronic alcoholics with the etiological agent still active, it is very probable that the centrilobular fibrosis gradually progresses and participates in the splitting up of the lobules[63].

Centrilobular fibrosis, for example central hyaline sclerosis, may cause venous outflow block.

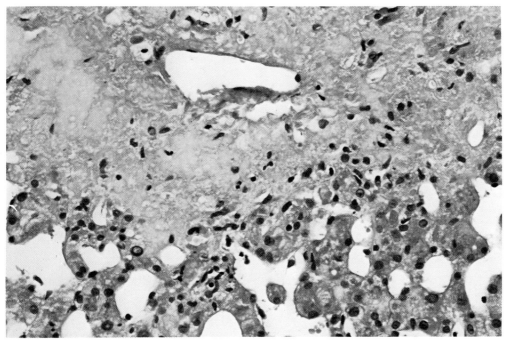

Fig. 148: Centrilobular area with central vein. At the bottom sinusoidal dilatation is seen, whereas the remaining part is fibrotic. Cardiogenic shock 6 months previously and at the time of biopsy a right-sided heart insufficiency (Needle biopsy, H & E x 270).

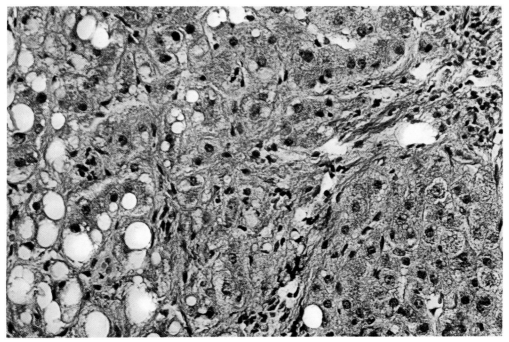

Fig. 149: Centrilobular area at lower left and part of a portal tract at upper right. Mainly in the centrilobular area irregular bundles of collagen fibers are salient, and a portal-central septum is also present. Chronic alcoholic (Needle biopsy, van Gieson x 270).

Bridging fibrosis

Morphology: Both in connection with periportal and with centrilobular fibrosis one often finds connective tissue extensions which stretch in the direction of other portal tracts or central veins. When the fibrous septa connect such structures they constitute bridging fibrosis[7], portal-portal when they connect portal tracts, portal-central when they connect portal tracts and central veins, and central-central when central veins are connected.

Portal-portal bridging fibrosis develop on the basis of liver cell necrosis comprising the part of the lobule which surrounds the terminal portal space. Portal-portal bridging thus represents a further development of the previously described periportal fibrosis with extensions in the direction of neighboring portal tracts. The location corresponds to the axis of Rappaport's acinus[300].

These septa can be present in varying sizes and shapes. Sometimes they are seen as relatively slender well-delimited bands which demarcate the individual lobule with a connective tissue membrane (Fig. 150).

Portal-central bridging fibrosis arises following bridging necrosis[40] (p. 90). The extent often corresponds mainly to the periphery of Rappaport's acinus[300]. The fibrotic septa are nearly always irregularly distributed throughout the lobules, and they are usually of varying breadth. In most instances there is inflammatory-cell infiltration in the connective tissue, sometimes slight and sometimes severe; as a rule the inflammation is most pronounced periportally and in the marginal areas close to the liver parenchyma (Fig. 151).

Central-central bridging fibrosis develops after confluent necrosis extending from a central vein of one lobule to the central vein of a neighboring lobule – so-called interlobular confluent necrosis[7]. Isolated central-central fibrosis is rare and is usually seen together with portal-central bridging fibrosis.

Morphological diagnosis: Prerequisites for an accurate diagnosis are: a large well-orientated and processed biopsy, sections stained for collagen fibers, and serial sections.

Differential diagnosis: As is the case with most other forms of fibrosis, the important differential diagnostic problem is between fibrosis and necrosis. Transitional forms between bridging necrosis and bridging fibrosis are met with, and staining for collagen fibers is necessary. Only when true fibrous septa are demonstrable may the lesions be called bridging fibrosis.

Additional morphological findings: Bridging fibrosis is most commonly seen in cases with severe acute hepatitis, in chronic aggressive hepatitis and in alcoholic liver disease, and the changes characteristic of these conditions are therefore likely to be present. Central-central bridging fibrosis arising after severe acute heart failure is in many instances associated with centrilobular and posibly intermediate sinusoidal dilatation.

Occurrence and significance: Slender portal-portal bridging fibrosis is relatively common in the late stages of acute hepatitis and is in our experience of no prognostic significance[101]. Broader portal-portal bridging fibrosis and portal-central bridging fibrosis is found in only a small porportion of patients with acute hepatitis in our material[265], but in approximately half of our biopsies showing chronic aggressive hepatitis[58]. The demonstration of these forms of bridging fibrosis is a very important prognostic sign and gives rise to a strong suspicion that cirrhosis is developing[101].

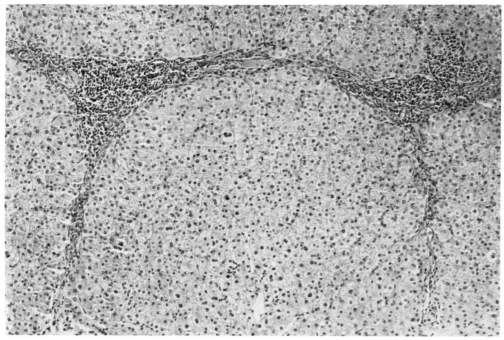

Fig. 150: Part of liver lobule (with central vein at bottom of the figure) with adjacent areas of three neighboring lobules. From a drug addict with a late stage of acute hepatitis. The patient made a complete recovery (Needle biopsy, van Gieson x 110).

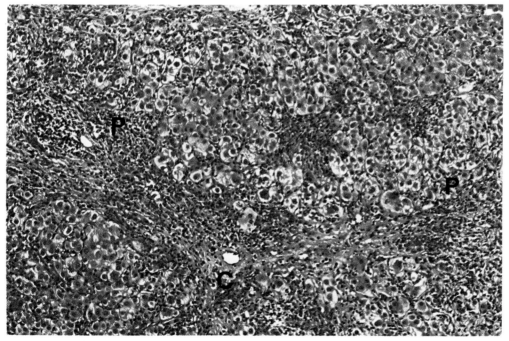

Fig. 151: Part of liver lobule with two portal tracts (P) and a central vein (C). Two broad septa are connecting the portal tracts with the central vein. From a patient with chronic aggressive hepatitis who developed cirrhosis (Needle biopsy, H & E x 110).

Panlobular fibrosis

Morphology: Panlobular fibrosis arises as a result of panlobular necrosis and may consequently vary in extent from a few lobules to the major part of the liver[274].

If a patient with panlobular necrosis (p. 88) survives for more than about a week, an increasing number of bile duct-like structures are seen mainly in the periphery of the necrotic lobule[274]. This is transformed into an area of collapse with preserved relationships between portal tracts and central veins, but with all distances reduced. Among the cells in this collapsed area are the perisinusoidal lipocytes or Ito cells, which are considered to be resting precursors of fibroblast, and it is probable that their stimulation accounts for some of the fibrogenesis which gradually changes the panlobular necrosis to an area of scar tissue, panlobular fibrosis[274].

In the early phases of panlobular fibrosis mild inflammation with a predominance of lymphocytes and histiocytes is virtually always present, but the inflammation is never severe and gradually diminishes.

Morphological diagnosis: The diagnosis is to be made on sections stained with H & E and sections stained for reticulin and collagen fibers. Prerequisites are collapse of whole lobules with diminished distances between portal tracts and central veins, complete or nearly complete lack of preserved liver cells and development of connective tissue corresponding to the original lobule (Fig. 152).

Panlobular fibrosis may involve the whole biopsy, and in such cases it is very important for the diagnosis that the original portal tracts and central veins should be identified in the large amounts of connective tissue present (Fig. 153). This is not always possible but depends to a high degree on the quality of the staining for collagen fibers. In our experience van Gieson's method is the most suitable.

Differential diagnosis: Staining for collagen fibers is necessary in the early stages for differentiation from panlobular necrosis.

Additional morphological findings: Panlobular fibrosis is found after rare cases of acute hepatitis induced by drugs[187, 272] or virus[96], and one may consequently see portal and parenchymal changes characteristic for the late stages of these conditions. Since panlobular necrosis may also arise at any time in the course of a chronic aggressive hepatitis[96], panlobular fibrosis can sometimes be found in biopsies showing this lesion (p. 176). Finally it should be mentioned that panlobular fibrosis is also a common finding in larger scars in cirrhosis[274].

Occurrence and significance: Panlobular fibrosis is recorded in less than 1 per cent of our liver biopsy material, and its presence is an expression of earlier, very severe parenchymal damage. Because of the usually uneven distribution the possibility of sampling error is high, and complete fibrosis of all lobules in a biopsy does not necessarily mean that the changes are widely disseminated throughout the liver. Conversly the absence of panlobular fibrosis in a biopsy does not signify that panlobular fibrosis is absent from other areas.

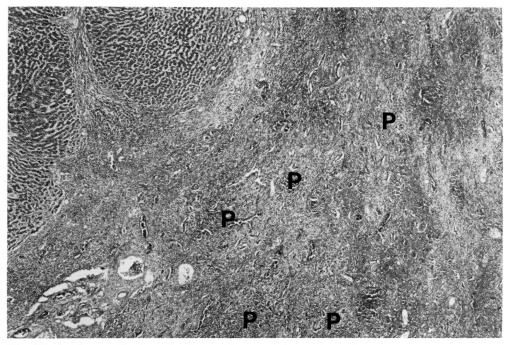

Fig. 152: Small magnification of a liver with extended panlobular fibrosis in which some portal tracts (P) with inflammation can be identified. In the upper left corner parts of two cirrhotic nodules are present. Posthepatitic cirrhosis (Surgical biopsy, H & E x 30).

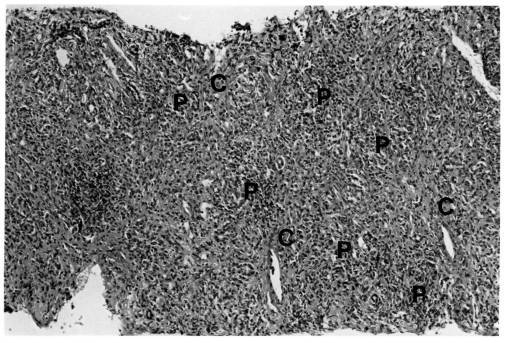

Fig. 153: Panlobular fibrosis comprising a number of lobules. The relationship between portal tracts (P) and central veins (C) is preserved but all distances are reduced. Posthepatitic cirrhosis (Needle biopsy, van Gieson x 110).

Fibrosis in cirrhosis

Morphology: By way of introduction it may be said that all the different forms of fibrosis in liver tissue with preserved lobular architecture discussed on the previous pages can be met with in cirrhotic livers. The lesions can not, however, always be identified as such; for instance, centrilobular and bridging fibrosis are often obscured during the reorganization of the liver architecture and by the continuous formation of new connective tissue.

In cirrhosis the parenchymal nodules are surrounded by connective tissue septa of varying breadth (Fig. 154). When the nodules are small and regular the fibrotic septa are often of a relatively uniform appearance from area to area, whereas in cirrhosis with nodules of varying sizes fibrous septa of varying breadth are usually found. Cirrhosis with large nodules and uniform, slender septa is called "septal cirrhosis"[274] (Fig. 155).

The increased amount of connective tissue in cirrhosis was previously regarded as being the result of collapse, but it is now thought to depend chiefly on active fibrogenesis[285]. New fibrous tissue is the result of fibroblast activity[285], but other cells, notably the fat-storing perisinusoidal cells of Ito, probably also participate[229]. The formation of fibers is often most prominent along the periphery of the acinus[285], thus producing portal-central bridging fibrosis. The collagen fibers in the newly formed septa are thin and loosely arranged. Gradually they are transformed to dense, more mature connective tissue. If the lesion is still active, inflammatory cells are found in the fibrous tissue and necrosis and inflammation are present in the adjacent parenchyma.

Morphological diagnosis: When the nodules are small, it is usually easy to demonstrate the fibrotic septa around individual nodules. In biopsies from cirrhotic livers with large parenchymal nodules difficulties often arise, but use of multiple sections in most cases discloses areas with increased amounts of connective tissue.

Differential diagnosis: Whereas sections stained for reticulin fibers are best for the recognition of parenchymal nodules, sections stained for collagen fibers are superior for the evaluation of the localization and degree of fibrosis. Without a collagen stain, collapse of the reticulin network may be misinterpreted as fibrosis. Furthermore, staining for collagen fibers often allows one to distinguish original portal tracts and central veins lying within the fibrous septa.

Additional morphological findings: Parenchymal nodules associated with fibrosis in a biopsy nearly always denote cirrhosis, and all the histological changes which may occur in cirrhosis are therefore to be found.

Occurrence and significance: Parenchymal nodules are most often diffusely distributed throughout the liver, and surrounded by connective tissue, a combination diagnostic for cirrhosis (see also p. 24).

Relatively uniform fibrotic septa in association with small nodules is often an expression of early cirrhosis and is most commonly found in alcoholics, whereas fibrous septa of varying breadth possibly with areas of panlobular fibrosis is more common in posthepatic cirrhosis. "Septal cirrhosis" is usually found in long-lasting and inactive cases[274].

Parenchymal nodules may also be seen in focal nodular hyperplasia. In this condition there are single or few localized lesions composed of nodules surrounded by connective tissue, with bile duct proliferation. A characteristic central scar with many vessels is usually found[111d] (p. 26).

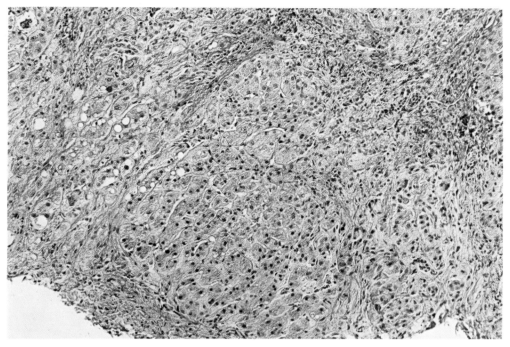

Fig. 154: Area of a micronodular cirrhosis with marked fibrosis. In the center two parenchymal nodules are seen, and on both sides are "incarcerated" small islands of liver cells (Needle biopsy, van Gieson x 110).

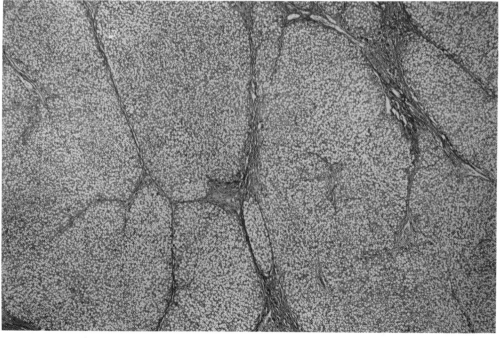

Fig. 155: Area of a macronodular cirrhosis with slender septa surrounding the nodules. There are no inflammation and liver cell necrosis to be found in this biopsy. From a patient who is now without symptoms from his cirrhosis (Surgical biopsy, H & E x 30).

Chapter III

Combination of Individual Features in Major Liver Diseases

Introduction

In chapter II emphasis was placed on a systematic description and illustration of the most common and significant individual morphological alterations or lesions found in liver biopsies mainly from adults.

Occasionally a diagnosis is established by the presence of a single and almost absolute criterion (Fig. 156) but in most cases pathological liver tissue presents a multitude of different lesions, and it is the task of the pathologist not only to recognize the individual lesions but also to combine and interpret them (Fig. 157).

It is not within the scope of this book to give a complete list and description of all liver diseases, and only a few of the more important ones are discussed in order to demonstrate how the combinations of the different individual lesions and their degree may give not only a morphological diagnosis of the actual disease but also information about severity and morphological activity and possibly also about etiology and prognosis.

In the choice of examples we have been guided by the major hepatic problems in which liver biopsy is important for establishing or confirming the diagnosis. These major problems can be summarized under the following headings.

1: **Liver biopsies in acute hepatitis:** An important use of liver biopsies is in diagnosing and following the progress of viral hepatitis and recognizing its complications. In this connection both chronic hepatitis, one of the complications of acute hepatitis, and non-specific reactive hepatitis and infectious mononucleosis are discussed as differential diagnostic possibilities.

2: **Liver biopsies in differentiation of causes of cholestasis:** In practice, the main causes to acute cholestasis to be distinguished are mechanical biliary obstruction, drug-induced cholestasis and acute viral hepatitis with cholestasis. The morphological changes in the first two and the differential diagnostic problems in relation to acute hepatitis with cholestasis are discussed. In addition a short description is given on primary biliary cirrhosis as a representative of a condition with a long lasting clinical cholestasis.

3: **Liver biopsies in cirrhosis:** The value of liver biopsy is not limited to diagnosis. Activity can be assessed by noting the degree of liver cell necrosis and inflammatory infiltration. It may be seen whether cirrhosis is well established, or whether the process appears to be at an early stage of development. In many cirrhotic biopsies there is histologic evidence of the etiology. Complications, notably liver-cell carcinoma, may be diagnosed. In this connection angiosarcoma is also described.

4: **Liver biopsies in congestive heart failure:** The majority of these patients are found to have hepatomegaly and, especially in acute heart failure the clinical picture may be indistinguishable from that of acute viral hepatitis. In this connection the differentiation from the Budd-Chiari syndrome and veno-occlusive disease are discussed.

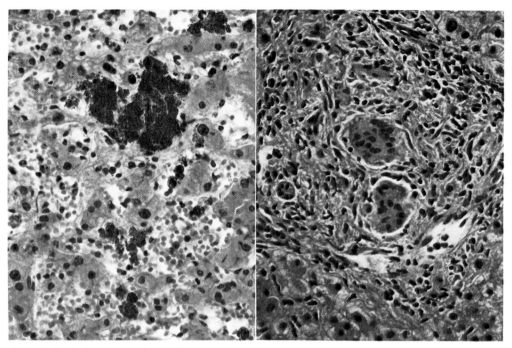

Fig. 156: Left. Thorotrast pigment in parenchyma, mainly localized in Kupffer cells (Needle biopsy, H & E x 270). Right. Portal tract with several multinucleated giant cells. Liver disease following treatment with phenyl butazone (Surgical biopsy, H & E x 270).

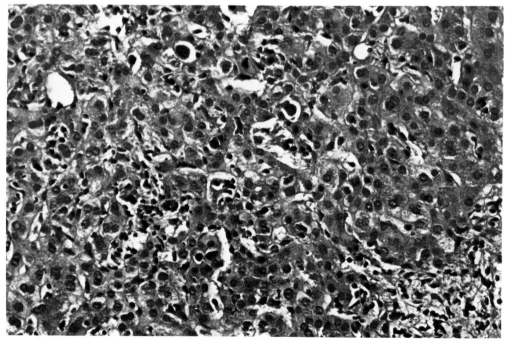

Fig. 157: Part of lobule with central vein (upper left) and portal tract (lower right): Changes such as focal liver cell necrosis, Kupffer cell proliferation, ballooning and portal inflammation indicate acute hepatitis. Cholestasis is pronounced (Needle biopsy, H & E x 270).

Acute, constant changes

Morphology: *Constant features:* focal liver cell necrosis, acidophil bodies, ballooning of liver cells, irregularity of liver cell plates, focal Kupffer cell proliferation, and portal inflammation (mainly lymphocytes, plasma cells and histiocytes)[29].

The so-called constant changes in acute hepatitis (syn. acute viral hepatitis) are found in virtually every lobule, although they vary in extent and intensity. The morphological pictures in the early, fully developed, late and residual stage differ to some degree[29, 96].

In the fully developed stage all the constant features are recognized both in the parenchyma and in all the poral tracts. The lobular changes are usually more pronounced in the centrilobular area than in other parts of the lobules (Fig. 158). If the morphological changes are mild they may be found only around the central veins[96]. The irregularity of the liver cell plates (Fig. 159) is mainly caused by focal necrosis, ballooning and rosette formation. In the earlier stages the parenchymal changes are usually more prominent than the portal ones, and a good marker for these stages is the presence of so-called ceroid pigment confined or nearly confined to intralobular histiocytes[28, 96]. In the fully developed stage the pigment is found in both intralobular and portal histiocytes, whereas in the later stages pigment is predominantly in portal tracts[29, 97].

The morphological changes vary not only with the course of the disease, but according to its severity they may also vary from one area of the same liver to another.

Morphological diagnosis: The diagnosis of acute hepatitis is based on the so-called constant changes, and is usually easy if the biopsy is adequate. When the changes are slight PAS staining after diastase is very helpful to reveal the ceroid pigment (Fig. 123).

Differential diagnosis: In cases with constant changes only differential diagnostic problems are usually small. When the morphological alterations are slight the picture may be difficult to distinguish from non-specific reactive hepatitis[34]. However, the amount of ceroid, the number of acidophil bodies and the degree of ballooning are virtually always greater in acute hepatitis[29].

Additional morphological findings: The constant changes may be followed by a series of inconstant changes. These are discussed on page 174.

Occurrence and significance: Most patients with the above changes have a hepatitis provoked by hepatitis virus, A, B or other types ("non A – non B"). No characteristic light microscopic differences between the different types have been described in man[29, 268].

The same morphological picture can be seen in liver injury after certain drugs (p. 184)[30, 187, 259, 272]. In many instances lesions such as granulomas, abnormal bile duct epithelium, inflammation with predominance of eosinophils, well-demarcated confluent necrosis or severe cholestasis raise a suspicion of a drug lesion but this is not always the case[30].

Exceptional cases of infectious mononucleosis may show similar features[29, 288] and a few patients with connective tissue diseases have been shown to present both clinically and morphologically with acute hepatitis[335].

A special problem is so-called "chronic lobular hepatitis"[271] which is a condition lasting for many months or even years, continuously exhibiting the morphological features of acute hepatitis without signs of chronicity. These cases are uncommon, as are patients with acute relapsing hepatitis.

Nearly all patients with acute hepatitis of the type described above show complete recovery within months[265].

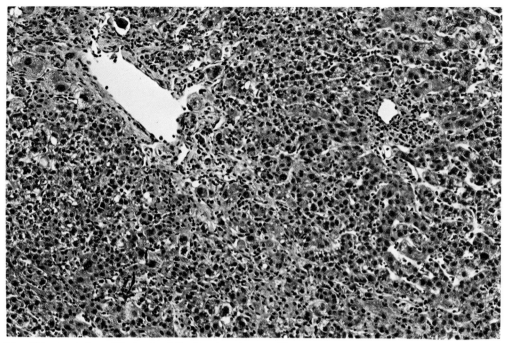

Fig. 158: Acute hepatitis in the fully developed stage. The parenchymal changes are severe with a centrilobular overweight. In the right side of the picture a small portal tract with only mild inflammation is seen (Needle biopsy, H & E x 110).

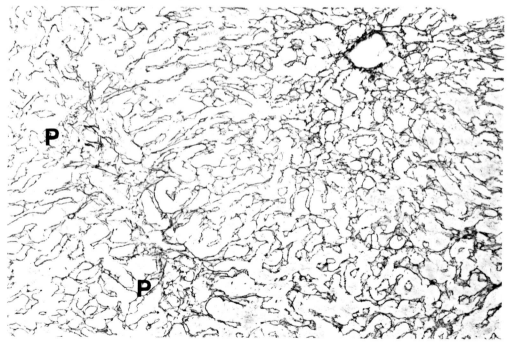

Fig. 159: From another case of acute viral hepatitis. The liver cell plates show a conspicuous irregularity mainly in the centrilobular zones (upper right). Portal tracts are indicated by P (Needle biopsy, reticulin x 110).

Acute, inconstant changes

Morphology: *Inconstant features:* iron in histiocytes, neutrophils in portal tracts, parenchymal cholestasis, fatty change, piecemeal necrosis, bile duct proliferation, abnormal bile duct epithelium, periportal fibrosis, confluent necrosis, bridging necrosis, panlobular necrosis, eosinophils in portal tracts and granulomas[29].

The inconstant changes which may be present in acute hepatitis, i.e. in addition to the constant changes, are seen with varying frequency. Iron in histiocytes, for instance is seen in approximately 50 per cent while granulomas are exceptional.

Morphological diagnosis: The diagnosis of acute hepatitis is normally made on the basis of the constant changes mentioned on the previous page. The morphological recognition of the individual inconstant lesions, is discussed in chapter II.

Differential diagnosis: Of special interest is the distinction between acute hepatitis with much piecemeal necrosis and chronic aggressive hepatitis with superimposed acute hepatitic changes. Of greatest importance is the periportal fibrosis, which constitutes a change mandatory for the diagnosis of chronic aggressive hepatitis[31]. The fibrosis in this disease is substantial, whereas increase in connective tissue in acute hepatitis is absent or slight. Transitional forms exist, and the term acute hepatitis with possible transition to chronicity has been proposed for cases with constant features of acute hepatitis associated with severe piecemeal necrosis[31].

Another differential diagnostic problem is cirrhosis. In cases with bridging necrosis the surviving parts of the parenchyma may form more or less rounded areas sometimes difficult to distinguish from nodules in cirrhosis, but serial sections stained with H & E and for reticulin will in most cases demonstrate that the destruction only comprises partial segmentation of lobules.

In a few cases of acute hepatitis there may be severe centrilobular cholestasis, many neutrophils and bile duct proliferation mainly in the marginal areas of the portal tracts and relatively modest liver cell damage[29,96]. This picture shows similarities to the changes found in large duct obstruction. As a rule the ballooning is more pronounced in acute hepatitis, and the amount of ceroid (and sometimes iron) in histiocytes is greater.

Additional morphological findings: Acute hepatitis is hardly ever associated with other lesions than those mentioned above. We have observed rare cases of acute hepatitis superimposed on cirrhosis and also, exceptionally, together with other changes such as alcoholic hepatitis. Orcein-positive ground glass cells have so far only been demonstrated in a few cases of acute hepatitis B with suspicion of transition to chronic hepatitis[32].

Occurrence and significance: Iron in histiocytes in our material of acute hepatitis cases is noted in approximately 50 per cent. The finding is of diagnostic importance but is probably of no prognostic significance[265].

Slight piecemeal necrosis is a common finding in acute hepatitis, whereas severe piecemeal necrosis is only present in a few per cent[265] (Fig. 160). The former is of no prognostic importance but the latter seems in the majority of cases to be followed by chronic aggressive hepatitis[31].

Areas of confluent necrosis are present in less than 10 per cent[265] (Fig. 161). Most of them are small and without prognostic significance. Larger areas – without concomitant piecemeal necrosis – may lead to fibrosis but probably not to cirrhosis[29]. For massive necrosis see p. 88.

Portal-central bridging necrosis comprising both piecemeal and confluent necrosis is, however, a sinister sign, and cirrhosis develops in many such cases[40,58].

Severe cholestasis is usually found in patients with a prolonged course of the disease, but it is an exception to see development of chronic hepatitis or cirrhosis[29,95] (Fig. 157).

Whether only constant or both constant and inconstant changes are seen in acute hepatitis, the possibility of etiological factors other than hepatitis viruses should always be kept in mind[29,30,187].

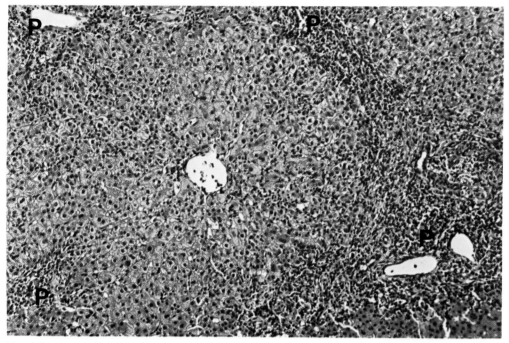

Fig. 160: Acute viral hepatitis with possible transition to chronicity. There is moderate to severe piecemeal necrosis but stain for collagen fibers discloses only minimal increase in the amount of connective tissue (Needle biopsy, H & E x 110).

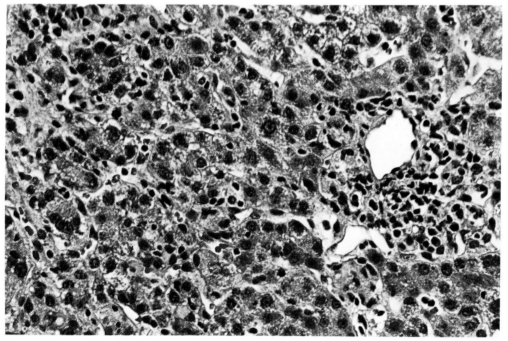

Fig. 161: Acute viral hepatitis with centrilobular area left and portal tract right. The liver cells in the left side are small with basophilic cytoplasm representing regeneration following centrilobular confluent necrosis (Needle biopsy, H & E x 270).

Chronic aggressive

Morphology: *Constant features:* periportal fibrosis, portal inflammation, piecemeal necrosis, non-specific hepatitis[40,89].
Inconstant features: changes as in acute hepatitis (both constant and inconstant features).

The lobular architecture is in milder cases preserved and in severe cases it is often somewhat irregular because of bridging fibrosis (Fig. 162) and bridging necrosis (Fig. 163)[89,307]. Transitional stages to cirrhosis are not uncommon[31]. The periportal fibrosis is of varying extent and uneven distribution but all in all the fibrosis is moderate to severe. An increased number of small bile ducts in the newly formed connective tissue is a constant finding. The degree of piecemeal necrosis also varies, not only from case to case but also from lobule to lobule[89,280].

Except for the periportal lesions the parenchymal changes are often mild, with only slight focal liver cell necrosis, slight focal infiltration with lymphocytes and histiocytes and possibly a few fat droplets.

In some cases the picture of acute hepatitis may be superimposed[89]. This implies that all the constant and inconstant findings which may arise in relation to this disease can be met with (p. 172 and p. 174). Of the inconstant features confluent necrosis[58], abnormal bile duct epithelium[59] and orcein-positive ground glass cells are common[32].

Morphological diagnosis: The diagnosis is to be made on H & E-stained sections and sections stained for collagen and reticulin fibers. It is necessary to use many sections in order to elucidate the architecture carefully.

Differential diagnosis: Sometimes biopsies in some areas show chronic aggressive hepatitis and in other areas cirrhosis. Such cases are usually termed cirrhosis with chronic aggressive hepatitis[31]. A differential diagnostic problem may arise when chronic aggressive hepatitis with superimposed acute hepatitis resembles acute hepatitis with signs of possible transition to chronicity[31,89]. Conspicuous periportal fibrosis with accompanying bile duct proliferation indicates chronic hepatitis.

Primary biliary cirrhosis, particularly in its early stages, may in some instances resemble chronic aggressive hepatitis, but as a rule the piecemeal necrosis is less pronounced and the inflammation of the portal tracts less extensive[69,93]. The abnormality of the bile duct epithelium is furthermore usually of more destructive nature and often accompanied by granulomas[69].

Additional morphological findings: As indicated above, cirrhosis may also be present.

Occurrence and significance: Chronic aggressive hepatitis is diagnosed in approximately 1 per cent of our biopsies[59]. It is most often discovered in females in the fourth to seventh decade but is not uncommon in other age groups and in males[58].

The histological diagnosis as defined above – reached without knowledge of clinical data – has in our material always been made in patients with clinical and biochemical signs of parenchymal liver damage of more than 3 months duration (chronic active hepatitis)[58]. Most patients (approximately ½–⅔) develop cirrhosis[99]. Severe bridging necrosis and occurrence of abnormal bile duct epithelium point to a rapid conversion into cirrhosis[58,290].

In other patients the progression is slower, and both the clinical and the morphological picture may fluctuate with shorter or longer periods when the changes are those of chronic persistent hepatitis[58,382]. However, most of these patients eventually develop cirrhosis[99].

Many cases of chronic aggressive hepatitis develop from an acute hepatitis but some have an insidious onset[99]. The etiology is virus (often hepatitis B), drugs (e.g. oxyphenisatin, methyl dopa), or unknown[15,99]. Immunological alterations have been suggested, but are possibly a consequence of the liver disease and not the cause of it[240,276,278,341]. Recently alcohol has been suggested as a possible agent.

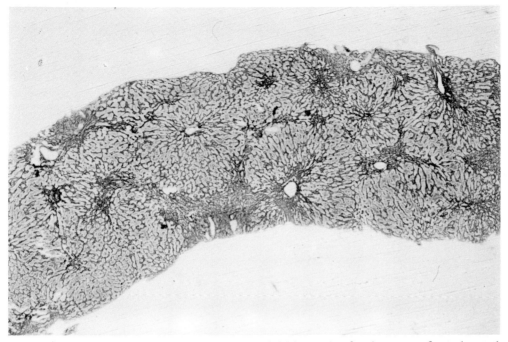

Fig. 162: Chronic aggressive hepatitis. Portal-portal bridging and a few instances of portal-central bridging are present. Van Gieson-stained sections showed that the septa were bridging fibrosis. No nodules (Needle biopsy, reticulin x 30).

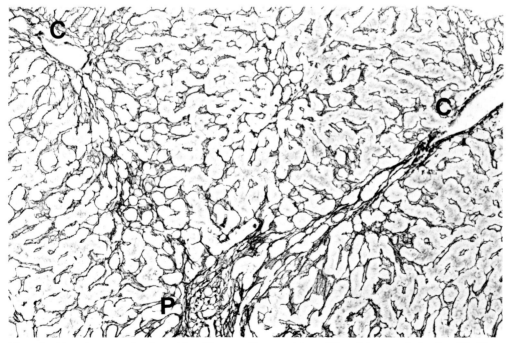

Fig. 163: Chronic aggressive hepatitis with part of a portal tract (P) and two central veins (C). Fine collapse of the reticulin framework corresponding to portal-central bridging necrosis is seen in both sides (Needle biopsy, reticulin x 110).

Chronic persistent

Morphology: *Constant features:* preserved lobular architecture, severe portal inflammation, non-specific reactive hepatitis[89,380].
Inconstant features: changes as in acute hepatitis (both constant and inconstant features).

The morphological picture is characterized by preserved lobular architecture and pronounced portal inflammation with predominance of lymphocytes and histiocytes but without or with only slight piecemeal necrosis, periportal fibrosis and bile duct proliferation[89,93,330]. In other words the limiting plate is preserved or only minimally destroyed (Fig. 164 & 165).

For this diagnosis to be made the inflammation must be pronounced and present in a substantial proportion of portal tracts. Often a few portal tracts show only slight or even no inflammation.

The lobules in most cases show only slight or minimal changes with focal liver cell necrosis and focal infiltration of lymphocytes and histiocytes. Orcein-positive ground glass cells are common. Changes as seen in acute hepatitis may be superimposed[31,89].

Morphological diagnosis: The morphological picture is non-specific, and the diagnosis can only be made by combining both clinical and morphological findings[89,93,208]. The clinical basis is longstanding evidence of parenchymal liver damage[98] (more than 3 or 6 months depending on the definition).

Differential diagnosis: The biggest problem is distinction from so-called non-specific reactive hepatitis with severe portal inflammation[89,208,319]. The latter is seen mainly in diseases of the organs drained by the portal vein and especially in relation to chronic peptic ulcer, chronic pancreatitis and chronic cholecystitis. The picture may be indistinguishable from chronic persistent hepatitis and the diagnosis depends on the clinical findings[98].

Chronic persistent hepatitis with superimposed acute viral hepatitis may be difficult to distinguish from acute hepatitis or chronic lobular hepatitis (p. 172). The presence of portal inflammation of unusual intensity and, if present, orcein-positive ground glass cells may give the correct diagnosis of chronic persistent hepatitis, but most often it is not possible to make this without clinical information.

Chronic persistent hepatitis with scattered piecemeal necrosis and mild to moderate periportal fibrosis may be difficult to distinguish from mild chronic aggressive hepatitis. Serial sections usually gives the answer, but is has to be stressed that follow up biopsies from some patients may reveal alternating chronic persistent and chronic aggressive hepatitis[58,353]. The appropriate diagnosis is then chronic aggressive hepatitis.

For a differentiation from malignant lymphoma, see p. 62.

Additional morphological findings: Inconstant changes, as found in some cases of acute hepatitis, may be present, but these are usually only slight. Examples are steatosis, cholestasis, confluent necrosis and abnormal bile duct epithelium[58].

Occurrence and significance: Chronic persistent hepatitis is less common than chronic aggressive hepatitis; 80–90 per cent have an acute onset and approximately 50 per cent are HB_SAg positive. Most arise in the second and third decade but all ages are represented. In the younger age groups there is a preponderance of males (drug addicts), in the older, females[98].

Presence of orcein-positive ground glass cells and sanded nuclei speaks in favor of a hepatitis B virus etiology, and large numbers of sanded nuclei, especially seen in biopsies from renal transplant recipients, indicate immunosuppression.

Chronic persistent hepatitis is an immunologically heterogeneous group. It may last for many years but the prognosis is generally good, and only in very few patients cirrhosis develops[98].

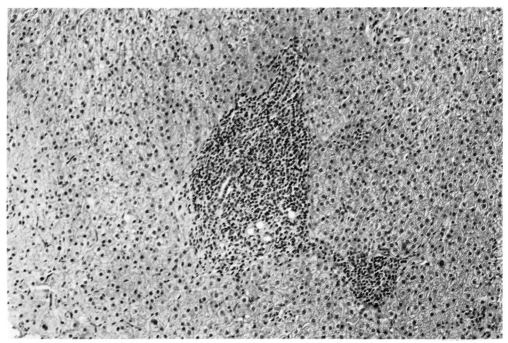

Fig. 164: Chronic persistent hepatitis. In both the portal tracts there is a dense inflammatory infiltrate with mononuclear cells. The limiting plate is preserved and only minimal changes are present in the parenchyma (Needle biopsy, H & E x 110).

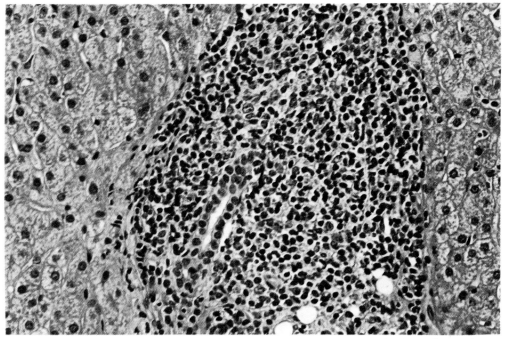

Fig. 165: Chronic persistent hepatitis. Higher magnification of the medium-sized portal tract shown above. Both lymphocytes, plasma cells and histiocytes can be identified. No bile duct proliferation (Needle biopsy, H & E x 270).

Non-specific, reactive

Morphology: *Constant features:* preserved lobular architecture, focal liver cell necrosis, focal Kupffer cell proliferation, slight portal infiltration with lymphocytes and histiocytes[29,208,319] (Fig. 166 & 167).
Inconstant features: acidophil bodies, steatosis, infiltration with neutrophils and plasma cells, lymphoid follicles in portal tracts.

In so-called non-specific reactive hepatitis one finds widespread portal and parenchymal changes in liver tissue with preserved lobular architecture. The portal tracts are typically infiltrated mainly by lymphocytes and histiocytes. The inflammation is irregularly distributed, and as a rule some tracts are normal whereas others show slight to moderate cellular infiltration. Often there are also a few neutrophils, eosinophils and plasma cells, and in exceptional cases lymphoid follicles may be present. The limiting plate is preserved and there is no fibrosis.

In the parenchyma focal liver cell necrosis and focal inflammation are characteristic. The number of necrotic lesions is usually small. They are irregularly distributed and most often of varying size and shape. They are accompanied by lymphocytes and histiocytes, the latter without or with only small amounts of pigment. One may find slight inflammation in some areas of the parenchyma without liver cell necrosis but serial sections show that this is rare; a few acidophil bodies are virtually always demonstrable.

Slight steatosis is common and in many such cases a small number of small lipogranulomas is present.

The literature suggests that portal and parenchymal inflammation as described above may be found independently[319]. In our experience, with use of routine serial sections, this is virtually never the case.

In addition to the above-mentioned diffuse form, which is widespread in the liver, non-specific reactive hepatitis can also be local, mainly in relation to metastases.

Morphological diagnosis: The diagnosis is best made on H & E-stained sections and at relatively small magnifications.

Differential diagnosis: The diagnosis is in most cases easy but sometimes the picture may be difficult or even impossible to distinguish from acute hepatitis (in the late or residual stages), chronic persistent hepatitis or infectious mononucleosis. In acute hepatitis the outline of the areas of liver cell necrosis is as a rule more rounded and the histiocytes contain more ceroid. There are also more necroses in acute hepatitis and more variation is seen in the size of the liver cells and the liver cell nuclei. The presence of bile thrombi speaks in favor of acute hepatitis, whereas steatosis, which is only rarely seen in acute hepatitis but in more than half of cases of non-specific reactive hepatitis, is in favor of the latter.

In the minority of biopsies with severely inflamed portal tracts, the picture may be indistinguishable from chronic persistent hepatitis (p. 178).

Additional morphological findings: Epithelioid cell granulomas, as found, for instance in sarcoidosis and miliary tuberculosis, are accompanied by changes of the non-specific reactive hepatitis type. Such changes may also be superimposed on a cirrhosis.

Occurrence and significance: The diffuse form of non-specific reactive hepatitis is found in approximately 5–10 per cent of our material and is seen in biopsies from patients either with more or less generalized diseases or with disorders in organs drained by the portal vein. Examples of the former are connective tissue disorders (especially rheumatoid arthritis)[100], influenza, sarcoidosis[190] and severe pneumonia[402], and examples of the latter include chronic peptic ulcer, cholecystitis, pancreatitis, ulcerative colitis[45,89,109], Crohn's disease and cancer of the stomach, bowel and pancreas. Drugs may also provoke a similar picture.

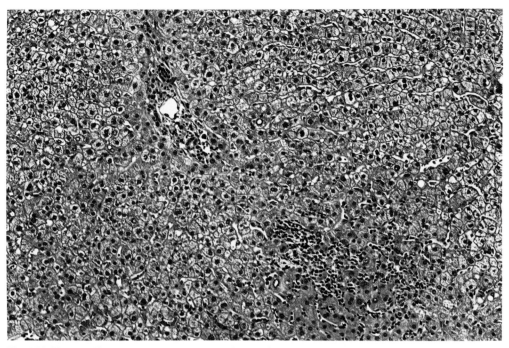

Fig. 166: Nonspecific reactive hepatitis with a few irregular and irregularly distributed lesions of focal liver cell necrosis and focal Kupffer cell proliferation. A very slight portal inflammation is also recognizable (Needle biopsy, H & E x 110).

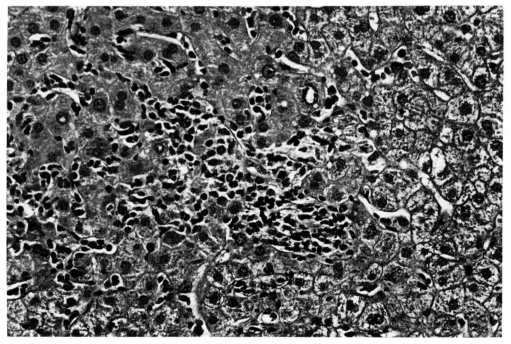

Fig. 167: Same area as Fig. 166. The typical focal necrosis of nonspecific reactive hepatitis differs mainly from the focal necrosis of acute hepatitis by its irregular form and by complete or nearly complete lack of ceroid pigment (Needle biopsy, H & E x 270).

Infectious mononucleosis

Morphology: *Constant features:* preserved lobular architecture, parenchymal and portal infiltration with mononuclear cells[17,29,188,387].
Inconstant features: focal liver cell necrosis, scattered plasma cells, acidophil bodies, cholestasis, steatosis, liver cell mitoses.

The mesenchymal reaction in the portal tracts is dense and comprises virtually only large monocytoid cells with basophilic cytoplasm and often with indented nuclei. The infiltration may spread to the adjacent parts of the parenchyma both in the form of spill-over and in relation to periportal liver cell necrosis. Scattered plasma cells may be found[24,188] (Fig. 168).

In the parenchyma one finds cells similar to those in the portal tracts. The infiltrates comprise two types of which one is seen as small rounded or irregular accumulations often in close relation to focal liver cell necrosis. The other, more characteristic type is more diffuse with poorly delimited aggregates along the sinusoids often involving large parts of the lobules (Fig. 120 & 169). The cells contain little or no ceroid.

In infectious mononucleosis the cellular infiltration is more prominent than parenchymal cell necrosis. A few acidophil bodies are virtually always to be found but there is as a rule no substantial variation in the size and shape of the liver cells and the liver cell nuclei. After some time liver cell mitoses are usually to be found in every lobule. The reticulin network is preserved[188].

Morphological diagnosis: The diagnosis is best made on H & E-stained sections and based on the relatively severe mesenchymal reaction both in portal tracts and parenchyma, dominated by monocytoid cells with indented nuclei and basophilic cytoplasm. In addition it is essential for the diagnosis that both focal and diffuse infiltrates should be present in the parenchyma.

Differential diagnosis: The picture is sometimes so typical that no differential diagnostic problems arise. At other times it may, however, be difficult or even impossible to distinguish infectious mononucleosis from acute hepatitis or nonspecific reactive hepatitis.

Infectious mononucleosis differs from acute hepatitis in having a severe mesenchymal reaction in combination with only slight liver cell damage, by more dense infiltrates dominated by monocytoid cells and by a complete or nearly complete lack of ceroid. In addition many mitoses per lobule and lack of zonal distribution speaks in favor of mononucleosis[188].

The morphological picture of infectious mononucleosis differs from non-specific reactive hepatitis in the more pronounced and denser mesenchymal reaction with monocytoid cells and relatively few foci of liver cell necrosis.

The portal and parenchymal cellular infiltrates seen in infectious mononucleosis may be reminiscent of leukemia or malignant lymphoma (p. 62 & 140).

Additional morphological findings: Bile thrombi and fat vacuoles are demonstrable in a minority of cases.

Occurrence and significance: The liver is affected in more than 75 per cent of cases of infectious mononucleosis but only about 10 per cent have jaundice. The disease is most typically seen in adolescents and young adults[24,188].

Liver biopsy is of importance in patients who are clinically uncharacteristic and when the diagnosis is in doubt.

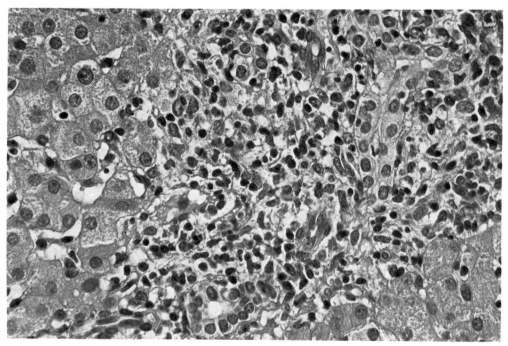

Fig. 168: Infectious mononucleosis. Portal tract with marked infiltration by mononuclear cells relatively rich in cytoplasm. Some nuclei are small and dark, others are larger with a looser structure. A few plasma cells can be seen (Needle biopsy, H & E x 270).

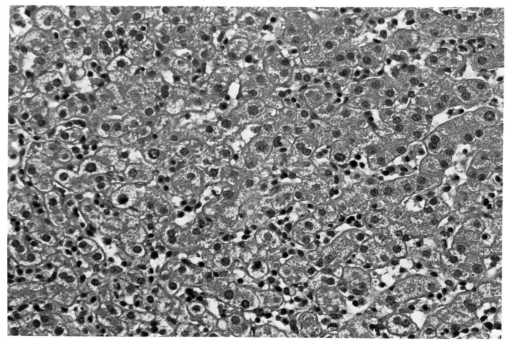

Fig. 169: Infectious mononucleosis. Part of a lobule with diffuse prominence and proliferation of cells along the sinusoids. Some of these cells have abundant cytoplasm (Needle biopsy, H & E x 110).

Drug-induced

Morphology: *Constant features:* preserved lobular architecture, bile thrombi in canaliculi.
Inconstant features: changes as in acute hepatitis, non-specific reactive hepatitis.

Drug-induced cholestasis may present a spectrum of morphological pictures from pure cholestasis, through cholestasis with slight to moderate parenchymal and portal changes, to cholestasis with a picture indistinguishable from acute viral hepatitis[30,187,259,272].

"Pure" cholestasis is defined as a lesion with morphological cholestasis without other changes such as liver cell damage and inflammation. Such a picture is mainly to be found as an early lesion (Fig. 60) and often focal liver cell necrosis and Kupffer cell proliferation supervene when the cholestasis has lasted for some days (Fig. 65). These changes are characteristically seen around bile thrombi.

In cases with slight liver cell damage one finds focal necrosis and variation in size of cells and nuclei. Focal infiltration with lymphocytes and Kupffer cells is also present and there is usually slight portal inflammation with lymphocytic predominance and sometimes many eosinophils. The parenchymal changes are usually most pronounced in the centrilobular zone and the picture could be termed "cholestasis with acute hepatitis grade ½" (Fig. 170).

In cases with a picture indistinguishable from acute viral hepatitis, the constant features of acute hepatitis are often accompanied by some of the inconstant features (p. 174) (Fig. 171). Following halothane there is most often a sharp demarcation of areas of confluent necrosis from non-necrotic parenchyma.

Morphological diagnosis: The recognition of bile thrombi is best made in sections stained for iron or with van Gieson.

Differential diagnosis: In cases with "pure" cholestasis the chief problem is the differentiation of the lesion from biliary obstruction. An adequate biopsy with many portal tracts lacking the characteristic changes (p. 186) excludes large duct obstruction[291].

In cases with mild to moderate reaction in the parenchyma and in the portal tracts, and especially in cases with a picture of acute hepatitis, it may be difficult or impossible to distinguish drug-induced from virus-induced hepatitis on morphological grounds alone. The discrepancy between the degree of cholestasis and the degree of acute hepatitis, however, often allows a correct diagnosis to be made. Other important markers of drug etiology are eosinophilia, granulomas, steatosis and abnormal bile duct epithelium[30,187].

Additional morphological findings: In cholestasis with slight parenchymal changes the portal tracts are as a rule normal or only mildly inflamed, lymphocytes predominating. Exceptionally, however, edema and marginal bile duct proliferation are seen and sometimes the infiltrate includes many neutrophils. In such cases the distinction between parenchymal cholestasis and large duct obstruction may be difficult (p. 186).

Occurrence and significance: "Pure" cholestasis is uncommon. Most of our biopsies are from patients treated with steroids (17-ketosteroids, contraceptive pills, etc.)[322] but it is also to be found in relation to other drugs (e.g. chlorpromazine[401], methyldopa[257] or even halothane[192]) and other conditions such as recurrent intrahepatic cholestasis, cholestasis following severe infections, postoperative intrahepatic cholestasis and cholestatic jaundice of pregnancy.

Cholestasis with mild inflammatory changes is typically seen after chlorpromazine[401] but may also follow several other drugs[187,272]. The general rule is that a single drug is in most cases associated with one morphological picture but in a minority of cases may show a different one. For instance chlorpromazine is usually followed by cholestasis with "acute hepatitis grade ½" but pure cholestasis and acute hepatitis, with or without cholestasis are also sometimes to be found. Similarly halothane, methyldopa and isoniazid most often provoke an acute hepatitis picture but both cholestasis with mild inflammation and pure cholestasis have been found.

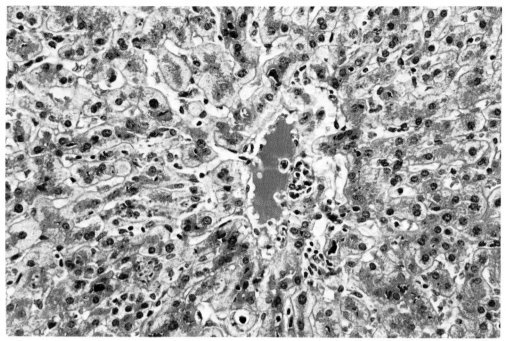

Fig. 170: "Cholestasis with acute hepatitis grade ½" following chlorpromazine. In addition to cholestasis some ballooning and slight focal liver cell necrosis and Kupffer cell proliferation are found (Needle biopsy, H & E x 270).

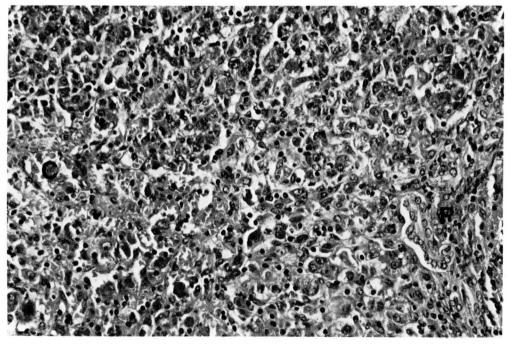

Fig. 171: Acute hepatitis with cholestasis following treatment with alpha-methyl dopa. Central vein left (C) and portal tract right (P). The parenchymal damage is severe with much focal liver cell necrosis and acidophil bodies (Needle biopsy, H & E x 110).

Large duct obstruction

Morphology: *Constant features:* cholestasis, marginal bile duct proliferation, edema of portal tracts, neutrophils in portal tracts[291].
Inconstant features: focal liver cell necrosis, periportal fibrosis, cirrhosis.

The combination of centrilobular cholestasis and portal changes with marginal bile duct proliferation, edema and infiltration of mainly neutrophils is characteristic for large duct obstruction[67, 291] (Fig. 172).

The cholestasis is initially centrilobular and not accompanied by liver cell damage or inflammation. Later both may develop but virtually always to a slight degree. The damage and the inflammation are most pronounced around bile thrombi. In cases with longstanding obstruction the cholestasis becomes more diffuse with bile thrombi also in the periportal parenchyma[291].

The marginal bile duct proliferation is the most constant of the portal lesions[138] but the others are nearly always present. However, not all portal tracts are involved in every case although as a rule most of them are[291]. In longstanding obstruction there may be destruction of the limiting plate with periportal fibrosis and later possibly secondary biliary cirrhosis (Fig. 173).

Morphological diagnosis: Sections stained with H & E and for iron, reticulin and collagen fibers are recommended. The diagnosis rests on the above-mentioned positive findings and the absence of other changes such as acute or chronic hepatitis, granulomas, piecemeal nerosis, lymphoid follicles or bile duct lesion.

Differential diagnosis: The series of changes characteristic of obstruction of large bile ducts is most typically seen in the first and second week after onset of jaundice. Later the liver cell damage and inflammation may imitate acute hepatitis. The amount of ceroid pigment is in general larger in acute hepatitis than in obstruction.

For distinction from drug lesions see p. 184).

Changes like those seen in large duct obstruction may also be found in some cases of primary biliary cirrhosis before the development of cirrhosis. The changes are found mainly in small portal tracts. Serial sections often disclose abnormal bile duct epithelium and possibly granulomas in larger tracts.

Additional morphological findings: The changes in question may be superimposed on a cirrhosis of any etiology, and in longstanding obstruction cirrhosis may develop.

It should be mentioned that the picture of large duct obstruction may also be seen in a more or less localized form in relation to focal lesions particularly around metastases.

Occurrence and significance: This type of cholestasis is called "large duct obstruction" and not "extrahepatic bile duct obstruction", because it is impossible on a biopsy alone to determine whether an obstruction e.g. by stone, inflammation or tumor is localized to the papilla of Vater, to the extrahepatic ducts or to the larger intrahepatic ducts.

A rather common cause is pancreatitis, probably most often an acute exacerbation of chronic disease. This is mainly seen in alcoholics with changes of large duct obstruction together with steatosis and alcoholic hepatitis, with or without cirrhosis[242]. One cannot in such cases exclude surgical correctable obstruction but usually the cholestasis gradually subsides after abstinence.

On the other hand the portal changes, in particular the marginal bile duct proliferation, are so constant a phenomenon, that if they are absent in an adequate biopsy with many portal tracts, large duct obstruction can be excluded[291].

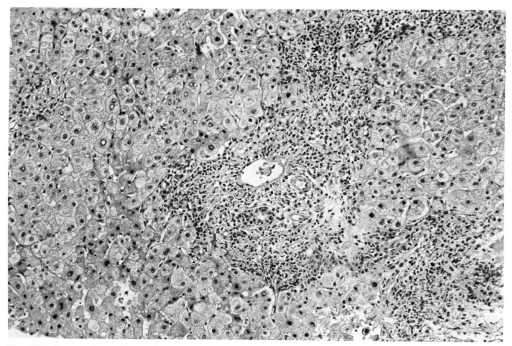

Fig. 172: Large duct obstruction of approximately 6 weeks duration. The centrally located portal tract shows a marked enlargement with inflammation, edema and bile duct proliferation mainly in the peripheral (marginal) parts of the tract (Needle biopsy, H & E x 110).

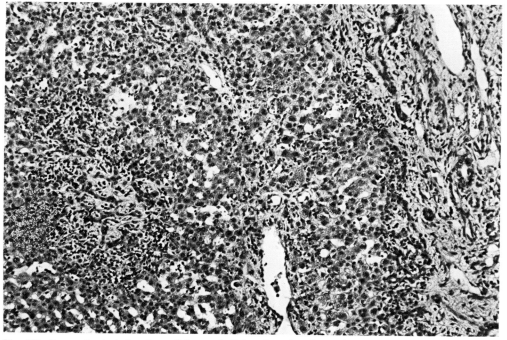

Fig. 173: Large duct obstruction of 9 months' duration showing enlarged portal tracts, destruction of the limiting plate and splitting up of the lobules. In other areas typical cirrhotic nodules were demonstrated (Surgical biopsy, H & E x 110).

Primary biliary cirrhosis

Morphology: *Constant features:* portal inflammation with abnormal interlobular and septal bile ducts, non-specific reactive hepatitis[93].

Inconstant features: granulomas, bile duct proliferation, orcein positive granules, fibrosis, cirrhosis, cholestasis, piecemeal necrosis, Mallory bodies[93].

The disease has on morphological criteria been divided into 4 stages, although considerable overlapping may occur[153, 279].

Stage 1 ("florid duct lesions") is characterized by having abnormal epithelium ("PBC-type") in segments of interlobular and septal bile ducts with inflammation and often granulomas (Fig. 44 & 45). The architecture is preserved (Fig. 174) but the limiting plate may be partly destroyed by piecemeal necrosis[153]. Cholestasis is rare, if present, it is centrilobular.

In stage 2 ("ductular proliferation") the affected bile ducts are destroyed and replaced by fibrotic tissue with inflammation (Fig. 34 & 35). Gradually irregularly distributed periportal fibrosis develops. Proliferation of marginally situated bile ducts is as a rule seen in some small and large portal tracts in both stage 1 and stage 2, just as the florid duct lesion often can be demonstrated in some tracts also in stage 2. Mainly periportal cholestasis and periportally located Mallory bodies may be found. Periportal orcein positive granules are very common.

Through stage 3 ("scarring") and stage 4 (cirrhosis) there is a gradual progression of the fibrosis, and only the last stage fulfills the definition of cirrhosis (Fig. 175). The changes of stage 1 and 2 can often be demonstrated in the later stages when multiple sections are used.

The term primary biliary cirrhosis is thus not logical, since cirrhosis is only present in stage 4, but it is generally accepted[325].

Morphological diagnosis: It is probably wise only to give a definite diagnosis of primary biliary cirrhosis when both typical abnormal epithelium and associated granuloma are present, or when multiple portal tracts contain characteristic scars with loss of original bile ducts. A strong suspicion of the diagnosis arises when either abnormal bile duct epithelium or granulomas are to be found, and also periportal orcein positive granules, cholestasis and Mallory bodies are weighty markers.

Non-specific changes found in a needle biopsy do not exclude a diagnosis of primary biliary cirrhosis, and surgical biopsies are superior to needle biopsies (p. 11). Multiple sections are of great diagnostic importance.

Differential diagnosis: An importal differential diagnostic problem is chronic aggressive hepatitis, and it is probable that the two conditions may be related; intermediate forms ("Zwischenformen") have been described[104]. As a rule the bile duct lesion in primary biliary cirrhosis shows traces of destruction and granulomatous reaction (p. 56), and in some cases cholestasis and Mallory bodies periportally, whereas typical signs of acute hepatitis are lacking[69].

Another important differential diagnostic problem is against large duct obstruction. As indicated above, changes as seen in obstruction of large bile ducts[291] may be found, and if the biopsy is not representative with regard to the lesions characteristic for primary biliary cirrhosis a wrong diagnosis can be made. This is especially probable with needle biopsies.

Additional morphological findings: Steatosis may be present, whereas a picture of acute viral hepatitis is absent.

Occurrence and significance: The diagnosis rests upon a combination of clinical (mainly middle-aged females, pruritus), biochemical (raised serum alkaline phosphatase and often high IgM and positive mitochondrial antibody test in serum) and morphological findings. The disease is associated with both humoral and cell mediated immunological disturbance, and some patients have in addition collagen disease and thyroiditis.

Presinusoidal portal hypertension frequently develops, and both hyperlipidemia and hypercholesterolemia often become prominent.

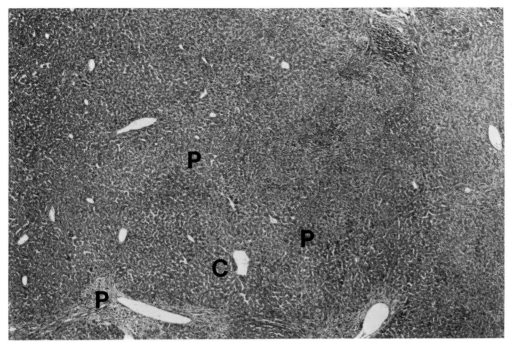

Fig. 174: Primary biliary cirrhosis, early stage without cirrhosis. In this small magnification one can see only inflammation in some portal tracts. Typical "florid duct lesion" has been demonstrated in the same biopsy (Surgical biopsy, H & E x 30).

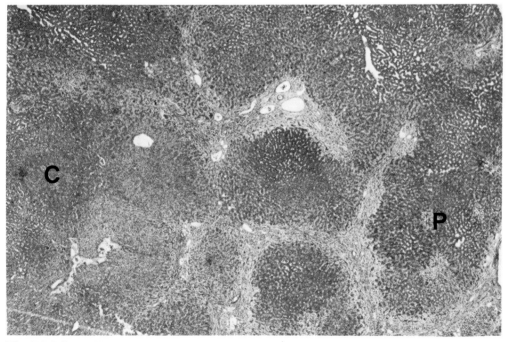

Fig. 175: Primary biliary cirrhosis, late stage with cirrhotic nodules and fibrosis. At higher magnification a marked decrease in the number of original bile ducts with scar formation was found (Surgical biopsy, H & E x 30).

Micronodular (regular)

Morphology: *Constant features:* widely distributed fibrosis associated with small, relatively uniform parenchymal nodules, bile duct proliferation[7,380].

Inconstant features: steatosis, alcoholic hepatitis, cholestasis, chronic aggressive hepatitis (both constant and inconstant features), changes as in large duct obstruction, abnormal bile duct epithelium, ("PBC" and "hepatitis" type), PAS-positive, diastase-resistant globules, siderosis, ischemic necrosis, dysplasia.

Cirrhotic nodules do not always develop simultaneously in all parts of the liver and all transitions between partly dissected lobules and fully developed nodules may be seen. A striking feature is the regularity of the nodule size. There are various definitions in the literature and limiting diameters of 1, 3 or 5 mm have been proposed. In our opinion 1 mm is the most suitable size on biopsy, especially needle biopsy. When the nodules are less than 1 mm, corresponding to the size of a normal lobule, the cirrhosis is termed micronodular[380]. There is a tendency for the micronodular pattern of cirrhosis to be seen relatively early in the course of cirrhosis and for larger nodules to develop later[364].

The degree of fibrosis may vary (Fig. 12, 154, 176 & 177) not only from patient to patient but also from one area to another in the same biopsy, but in the fully developed micronodular cirrhosis the fibrosis is most often rather evenly distributed throughout the liver.

Morphological diagnosis: The diagnosis of fully developed micronodular cirrhosis is virtually always easy, even though the biopsy is fragmented[43,326,388].

Differential diagnosis: In practice no problems arise in well-developed micronodular cirrhosis. It is probably wise to accept only biopsies with at least two complete nodules having fibrosis around the whole circumference as diagnostic.

Additional morphological findings: In micronodular cirrhosis the most common additional finding is steatosis and alcoholic hepatitis. A substantial number may, however, show chronic aggressive hepatitis in parts of the biopsy. PAS-positive, diastase-resistant globules and changes as in large duct obstruction are other, less common examples.

Occurrence and significance: Micronodular cirrhosis in our biopsy material is diagnosed in approximately 10 to 15 per cent of all cirrhosis cases. It is found in the early stages of most cirrhosis in chronic alcoholics and in many developing from chronic aggressive hepatitis. Primary and secondary biliary cirrhosis and cirrhosis in hemochromatosis and after passive congestion are also most often micronodular in the early stages[309].

The presence of partly preserved lobular architecture in cirrhotic tissue with an otherwise micronodular pattern is an expression of a cirrhosis at a very early stage[276,364]. Most such cases show in addition centrilobular hyaline sclerosis and alcoholic hepatitis[113]. We have so far only seen this combination (cirrhosis, partly preserved lobular architecture, micronodular pattern, centrilobular hyaline sclerosis, alcoholic hepatitis) in chronic alcoholics.

The picture of chronic aggressive hepatitis with micronodular cirrhosis is probably only seen in cirrhosis following chronic aggressive hepatitis. Cases with hepatitis B surface antigenemia often show ground glass changes[345], and the "PBC" type of abnormal epithelium in conjunction with granulomas gives the diagnosis of primary biliary cirrhosis[69,310].

A pattern with partly preserved lobular architecture is found in a high proportion of patients with relatively unusual conditions where the cirrhosis develops over a long period of time such as secondary biliary cirrhosis[103], some inborn errors of metabolism[167] and mucoviscidosis.

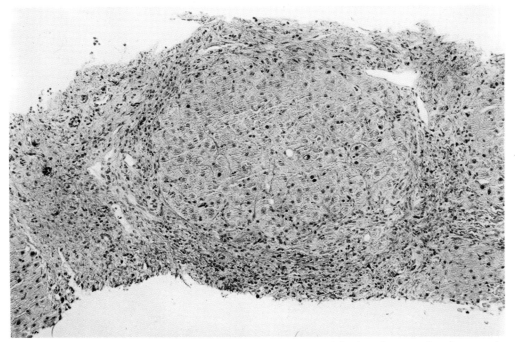

Fig. 176: Micronodular cirrhosis. A small nodule is surrounded by broad connective tissue septa with bile duct proliferation but only minimal inflammation. A few fat droplets are visible in the parenchyma. Chronic alcoholic (Needle biopsy, van Gieson x 110).

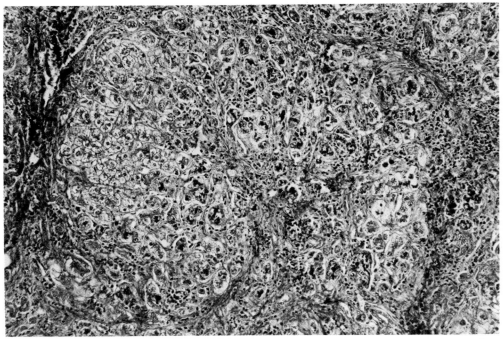

Fig. 177: Micronodular cirrhosis. The connective tissue septa are relatively slender. Many Mallory bodies are recognized in the liver cells which show marked variation in size and shape. Inflammation is slight. Indian childhood cirrhosis (Autopsy, Masson trichrome x 110).

Macronodular (irregular)

Morphology: *Constant features:* widely distributed fibrosis with parenchymal nodules of varying size, bile duct proliferation[7,380] (Fig. 178). *Inconstant features:* piecemeal necrosis, signs of hepatitis, steatosis, alcoholic hepatitis, cholestasis, abnormal bile duct epithelium, siderosis, ischemic necrosis, dysplasia.

When one or more nodules in a cirrhosis is larger than 1 mm, it is regarded as macronodular. Macronodules in macronodular cirrhosis may arise either primarily or secondarily, the latter by a gradually increasing size of micronodules[276,364]. Many of the larger nodules often contain portal structures and so-called efferent veins, although these are usually abnormally related to each other. The so-called efferent veins are in some instances preserved central veins, in others localized dilatations of the sinusoids. Some parts of macronodules may bear a close resemblance to normal liver tissue containing only slender septa of connective tissue. In other parts of the liver rounded nodules and broader fibrous septa are seen.

Morphological diagnosis: The diagnosis of macronodular cirrhosis is easy when small nodules are represented in the biopsy. More difficult and sometimes not diagnostic are cases with only parts of large nodules in the biopsied material[14,43,326,352,388]. Serial sections in combination with stains for reticulin and collagen fibers may be helpful.

A large surgical biopsy which is both deep and broad is in some cases superior to a needle biopsy.

Differential diagnosis: As mentioned in connection with micronodular cirrhosis the diagnosis cirrhosis is appropriate only when at least two complete nodules with surrounding fibrosis are present in the biopsy. In this way one will undoubtedly underdiagnose some cases but the possibility of overdiagnosis is minimal. A strong suspicion of cirrhosis is raised by the following: fibrous septa traversing the specimen, abnormal liver cell plates (p. 74), altered vascular relationship and fragmentation of the biopsy material.

Additional morphological findings: In macronodular cirrhosis the most common additional findings are piecemeal necrosis and signs of hepatitis, sometimes with confluent necrosis and collapse. All the inconstant features mentioned may be found. Steatosis, alcoholic hepatitis and cholestasis are relatively frequent, but less common than in micronodular cirrhosis. Many examples show no specific changes and often only slight or no histologic activity.

Occurrence and significance: As mentioned above, macronodules in macronodular cirrhosis may arise either primarily or secondarily, the latter by increasing size of micronodules. A primary macronodular cirrhosis is most commonly found in cases arising from acute or chronic aggressive hepatitis with severe and irregularly distributed confluent, bridging and panlobular necrosis.

It is sometimes noted that when the cirrhosis in such cases is fully developed the histological activity (liver cell damage and mesenchymal reaction) ceases with or without treatment, and in follow-up biopsies a histologically inactive cirrhosis with increasingly thinner connective tissue septa is found ("septal cirrhosis") (Fig. 13).

In alcoholics who stop drinking, features such as steatosis and alcoholic hepatitis usually disappear after approximately 1–2 months and 4–6 months, respectively[61]. The result after abstinence for a long period is often an inactive cirrhosis. Most types of cirrhosis are, as is the case in most alcoholics, micronodular in the early stages and macronodular in the later ones[276,364]. Examples are primary and secondary biliary cirrhosis and cirrhosis in hemochromatosis[309] (Fig. 179).

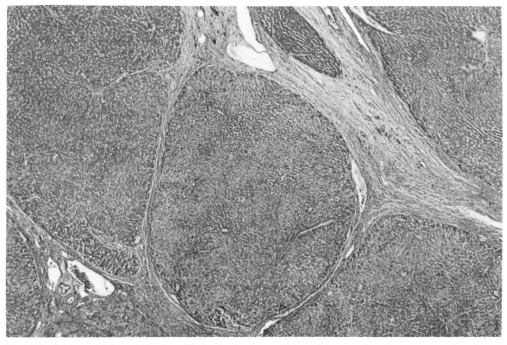

Fig. 178: Macronodular cirrhosis with both slender and broad connective tissue septa. One large nodule and parts of other nodules of varying sizes are seen. From a patient with Wilson's disease (Surgical biopsy, H & E x 30).

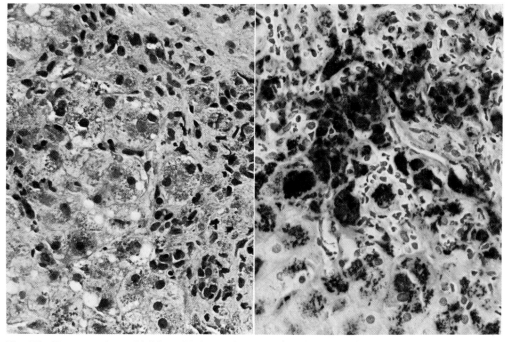

Fig. 179: From a patient with idiopathic hemochromatosis with macronodular cirrhosis. Left. Connective tissue and parenchyma with dispersed brown granules (H & E). Right. Same area with Perls' stain (Needle biopsy x 270).

Hepatocellular carcinoma

Morphology: *Constant features:* areas without lobular architecture; histological and cytological signs of malignancy (Fig. 180).
Inconstant features: In tumor cells: cholestasis, fat (Fig. 181), glycogen, Mallory bodies (Fig. 180), cytoplasmic or intranuclear globules. In non-neoplastic parenchyma: cirrhosis.

If a liver biopsy contains areas of hepatocellular carcinoma and areas of non-neoplastic liver tissue, the latter is usually cirrhotic[111d, 254]. Hepatocellular carcinomas are often trabecular, but may show areas partially simulating lobular architecture. It is important to note that portal tracts and bile ducts are missing, and that the tumor cells form plates of varying thickness and extent. Between the trabeculae, sinusoids and sometimes fibrous tissue are to be found, and in most cases very little or no reticulin can be demonstrated in the tumor tissue. Other forms of hepatocellular carcinoma are dominated by acinar structures, or they may be compact or scirrhous. All mixtures are described[3, 48, 84, 111d, 114, 136].

Tumor cells from a highly differentiated hepatocellular carcinoma may look very much like normal liver cells. It is, however, always possible to find cells with cytological signs of malignancy such as pleomorphism, hyperchromatism, enlarged nucleoli and increased numbers of mitoses. Abnormal mitoses may be seen. A special variant is a tumor predominantly or wholly composed of cells with clear cytoplasm (Fig. 181).

Poorly differentiated hepatocellular carcinomas always have an irregular architecture, and the tumor cells show conspicuous signs of malignancy sometimes with marked variation in cellular and nuclear size, shape and staining. In rare instances small or spindle-shaped tumor cells predominate.

Morphological diagnosis: It is usually easy to diagnose a moderately or well-differentiated hepatocellular carcinoma in H & E sections. The trabecular or acinar structure, the cytological signs of malignancy, and the invasion of the neighboring liver tissue are important and always sufficient criteria for the diagnosis. Bile and Mallory bodies have been reported only in

liver cell carcinomas and not in other carcinomas[111d]. Iron and lipofuscin are missing.

Poorly differentiated hepatocellular carcinomas are easily diagnosed as malignant epithelial tumors, but in some cases it is impossible to decide the origin.

Differential diagnosis: It may be difficult to distinguish highly differentiated hepatocellular carcinoma from cirrhotic nodules, and transitionel forms exist, so-called dysplasia[7].

Hepatocellular adenoma, an infrequently encoutered tumor, may also be difficult to differentiate from a well-differentiated hepatocellular carcinoma. The adenoma is formed by liver cells arranged in trabeculae – usually two or three cells thick. The architecture of the tumor tissue in areas often imitates the architecture of normal liver tissue, but portal tracts and bile ducts are absent, and only very few and dispersed arteries and veins can be demonstrated. The liver cells in an adenoma are larger than normal with large amounts of glycogen and sometimes fat and pigment (Fig. 110). There may be bile thrombi in the canaliculi. The nuclei are all of the same size with inconspicuous nucleoli. Areas of necrosis (Fig. 89) and hemorrhage are a common finding. The tumor is encircled by a capsule or delimited by a zone of compressed, non-tumorous liver tissue[19, 112, 189].

Cholangiocarcinoma is another candidate for diagnostic mistake. Presence of large amounts of connective tissue and lack of sinusoids, canaliculi and intracellular bile speak in favor of bile duct origin[48, 84, 111d, 114].

Additional morphological findings: Hepatocellular carcinoma is sometimes complicated by thrombosis of portal vein branches.

Occurrence and significance: Hepatocellular carcinoma has a worldwide distribution, but the incidence varies considerably[88, 117, 129, 140, 157]. In most countries hepatocellular carcinoma comprises only very few per cent of all cancers and usually arises in cirrhotic liver[243, 344, 364]. The overall prognosis is so far poor.

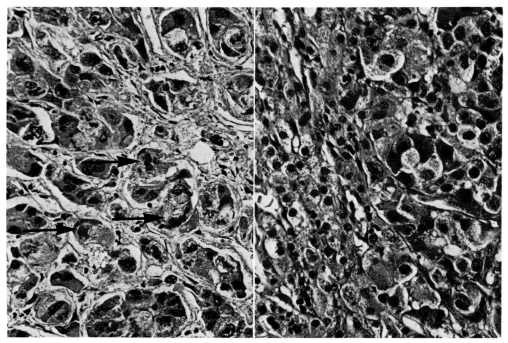

Fig. 180: Hepatocellular carcinoma. Left. Many of the tumor cells contain Mallory bodies (arrows). Right. The tumor cells are irregularly arranged and there are cytological signs of malignancy. The adjacent parenchyma is compressed (Autopsy, H & E x 270).

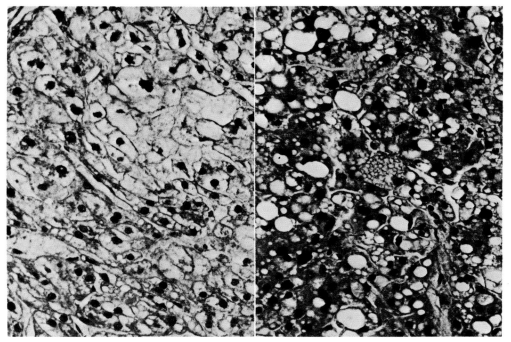

Fig. 181: Hepatocellular carcinoma. Left. From a tumor dominated by cells with clear cytoplasm. Right. Many of the tumor cells demonstrate fat vacuoles of varying size (Autopsy, H & E x 270).

Hemangiosarcoma

Morphology: *Constant features:* areas with destroyed architecture with proliferating angiomatous structures lined by cells with cytological features of malignancy, areas of necrosis and hemorrhage.

Inconstant features: cirrhosis, thorotrast pigment, liver cell necrosis, orcein-negative "ground glass" change, perisinusoidal fibrosis.

The malignant endothelial cells line blood-filled cavernous cavities (Fig. 182) and sinusoidal channels with areas of necrosis and hemorrhage. Solid areas are common. The cells are spheroidal and spindle-shaped with hyperchromatic and bizarre nuclei (Fig. 183). Multinucleate cells may be seen and mitoses are frequent[38, 47, 50, 196, 369]. Foci of hemopoiesis are often present. The malignant cells may be intimately related to liver cells and papillary or more solid structures may project into the vessels. The margins between the liver tissue and neoplastic tissue are irregular and indistinct with invasion of the liver along preexisting sinusoids and sometimes with tumor tissue growing into small veins. In other areas the liver parenchyma is compressed by tumor tissue, forming a "pseudocapsule".

Morphological diagnosis: The diagnosis is as a rule easy since relatively large amounts of tumor tissue with hemorrhagic necrosis usually are present. Proliferation and pleomorphism of sinusoidal cells may represent a premalignant state and may be found alone or in the marginal areas of frank hemangiosarcoma[369].

Differential diagnosis: Hemangiosarcomas are at times sufficiently similar to hemorrhagic hepatocellular carcinomas to cause confusion but in contrast to the latter they contain a rich network of reticulin fibers, and a reticulin staining together with multiple sections gives the right diagnosis.

Solid areas consisting of spindle cells are difficult to distinguish from fibrosarcoma but other characteristics such as growth into pre-existing vascular spaces are virtually always present.

Some problems may arise in connection with the so-called multiple hemangioendotheliomas seen in children[90]. The cytological signs of malignancy are the most important microscopic characteristics for distinguishing a sarcoma from a benign hemangioendothelioma.

Additional morphological findings: In some cases deposits of thorotrast in both neoplastic and non-neoplastic areas are demonstrable[161, 384]. In cases of angiosarcoma induced by PVC (polyvinyl chloride) the preserved liver tissue exhibits focal necrosis, focal adaptive changes in the cytoplasm of hepatocytes, enlargements of liver cells and pleomorphism of liver cell nuclei and a slowly progressive perisinusoidal fibrosis with proliferation of sinusoidal cells. Peliosis-like changes may also be found[369].

Thrombosis and areas of infarction are frequent and rupture of the liver may develop.

Occurrence and significance: Hepatic irradiation, such as exposure to thorotrast, is believed to be a predisposing factor[161, 384]. In recent years a relationship between PVC exposure and hemangiosarcoma of the liver has been reported[369]. The precise mechanism for the oncogenecity and hepatotoxicity of PVC is still unknown, but various experimental and clinical observations suggest that PVC, or some metabolic derivatives, presumably formed in the liver, affect both the hepatocytes and the sinusoidal lining cells.

Hemangiosarcomas of the liver most often affect adult males. They are highly malignant tumors and are usually rapidly fatal after discovery.

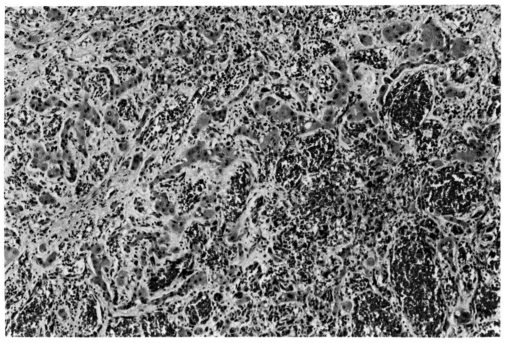

Fig. 182: Hemangiosarcoma with several large blood-filled spaces (mainly right) and many irregularly distributed, usually atrophic liver cell plates. Fibrosis is also present (Autopsy, H & E x 30).

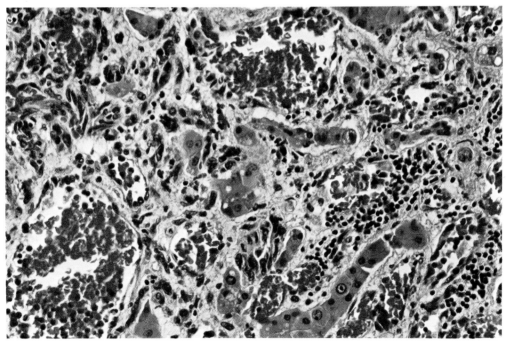

Fig. 183: Hemangiosarcoma, same specimen as Fig. 182. Both angiomatous formations and solid cords of tumor cell, some with hyperchromatic and bizarre nuclei, are seen. From PVC worker (Autopsy, H & E x 270).

Venous congestion

Morphology: *Constant features:* preserved lobular architecture, centrilobular dilatation of sinusoids, atrophy of liver cell plates.
Inconstant features: steatosis, cholestasis, centrilobular confluent necrosis, hemorrhage, central vein thrombosis.

Venous or passive congestion of the liver, most often met with in patients with right ventricular failure, may be found in an early or a late stage[52, 73, 338, 342]. In the early stages it is most common to see dilatation of central veins and centrilobular sinusoids with only slight atrophy of the liver cell plates. In the more severe cases centrilobular cholestasis is sometimes conspicuous and the picture may also be complicated by centrilobular confluent necrosis (with or without hemorrhage) and in very rare cases by central vein thrombosis[73, 342].

In the later stages of passive congestion the atrophy of the liver cell plates is more pronounced than in the early stages (Fig. 118) and commonly the changes also include the intermediate zone (Fig. 58). In the most severe cases even parts of the periportal zone are involved leaving only a small area around the portal tracts with non-atrophic liver cell plates and normal appearing sinusoids. Steatosis is found in many instances and mainly in the liver cells around the areas with constant changes. Slight fibrosis along the centrilobular sinusoids may rarely be demonstrated.

Centrilobular confluent necrosis (Fig. 184) and central vein thrombosis may arise at any stage of the development of the disease and all transitions from necrosis and thrombosis to fibrosis can be found[52, 338] (Fig. 185).

Morphological diagnosis: The constant changes are nearly always diagnosed with ease on H &E-stained sections (p. 70). The degree of fibrosis is best estimated on sections stained for collagen fibers.

Differential diagnosis: For constant changes see p. 79, inconstant changes p. 86 and p. 148.

Additional morphological findings: Nodular regenerative hyperplasia and so-called cardiac cirrhosis are very unusual pictures which may develop in longstanding and severe cases[360]. The latter is characterized by small nodules comprising rounded parts of the original lobules with portal-central septa and with atrophic liver cell plates and dilated sinusoids in relation to the original central veins, which can often be identified in sections stained for collagen fibers.

Venous congestion may also develop in cirrhotic patients. There is often dilatation of sinusoids and atrophy of liver cell plates but the lesions are as a rule less pronounced and without zonal distribution.

Occurrence and significance: The constant changes are most commonly found in patients with right-sided heart failure. A similar picture can, however, also be seen in biopsies from patients with chronic diseases with elevated serum globulin and low serum albumin[295].

Centrilobular necrosis with hemorrhage most often develops in connection with severe cardiac shock (of more than 24 hours' duration). If the patient survives the acute attack, a centrilobular fibrosis or, exceptionally, a cardiac cirrhosis may develop. Cardiac cirrhosis probably only develops in patients with severe cardiac shock followed by a long lasting and severe backward failure.

Centrilobular necrosis can also arise in patients with severe backward failure or be due to venous obstruction caused by, for instance, thrombosis or tumors. Both the Budd-Chiari syndrome (obstruction of the hepatic vein or its main branches)[86, 159] and VOD (thrombosis or fibrous occlusion of the central veins) are rare[42] (p. 148).

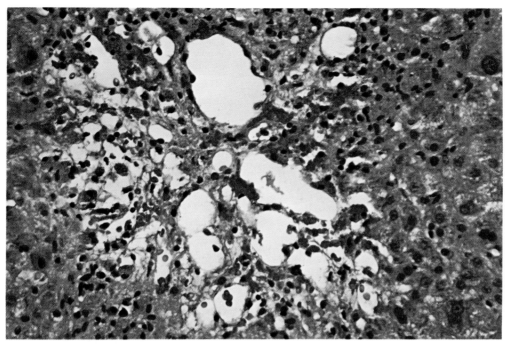

Fig. 184: Centrilobular confluent necrosis with small foci of hemorrhage. There is only minimal inflammation with a few mononuclear cells. 18 days after an acute myocardial infarction with cardiogenic shock (Needle biopsy, H & E x 270).

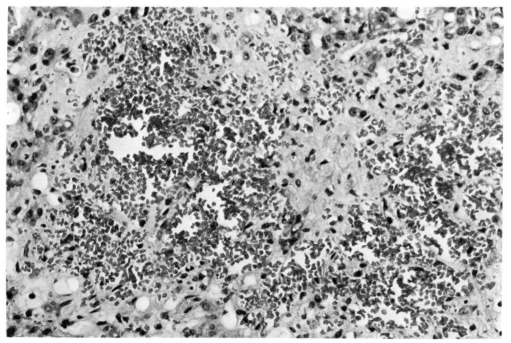

Fig. 185: Centrilobular area from a patient with a chronic Budd-Chiari syndrome. There are an extended network of anastomosing cords of loose connective tissue, hemorrhage and a few atrophic liver cell plates (Autopsy, H & E x 110).

References

1. *Abrahams, C., Wheatley, A., Rubenstein, A. H. & Stables, D.:* Hepatocellular lipofuscin after excessive ingestion of analgesics. Lancet *ii:* 621, 1964.

2. *Adams, D. O.:* The granulomatous inflammatory response. Am. J. Path. *84:* 164, 1976.

3. *Alpert, E., Uriel, J. & de Nechaud, B.:* Alpha-l-fetoprotein in the diagnosis of human hepatoma. N. Engl. J. Med. *278:* 984, 1968.

4. *Amos, J. A. S. & Goodbody, R. A.:* Lymph node and liver biopsy in the myeloproliferative disorders. Brit. J. Cancer *13:* 173, 1959.

5. *Andrade, Z. A.:* Hepatic schistosomiasis. In: Popper, H. & Schaffner, F. (ed.): Progress in Liver Diseases vol. 2. New York: Grune & Stratton. p. 228, 1965.

6. *Anthonisen, P., Christoffersen, P., Riis, P., Schourup, K.* & Schwartz, M.: Liver histology in ulcerative colitis. Acta med. scand. *180:* 551, 1966.

7. *Anthony, P. P., Ishak, K. G., Nayak, N. C., Poulsen, H., Scheuer, P. J. & Sobin, L. H.:* The morphology of cirrhosis. J. Clin. Path. *31:* 395, 1978.

8. *Antia, F. P., Bharadwaj, T. P., Watsa, M. C. & Master, J.:* Liver in normal pregnancy, pre-eclampsia and eclampsia. Lancet *ii:* 776, 1958.

9. *Ashkenazi, A., Yarom, R., Gutman, A., Abrahamov, A. & Russel, A.:* Niemann-Pick disease and giant cell transformation of the liver. Acta paediat. scand. *60:* 285, 1971.

10. *Aterman, K.:* Some observations on the sinusoidal cells of the liver. Acta Anat. *32:* 193, 1958.

11. *Aterman, K.:* The "dark" and the "light" cells of the liver. Anat. Rec. *136:* 157, 1960.

12. *Aterman, K.:* The structure of liver sinusoids and the sinusoidal cells. In: Rouiller, C. H. (ed.): The Liver: Morphology, Biochemistry, Physiology. vol. 1. New York: Academic Press p. 61, 1963.

13. *Baba, N. & Ruppert, R. D.:* The Dubin-Johnson syndrome: Electron microscopic observation of hepatic pigment, a case study. Am. J. Clin. Path. *57:* 306, 1972.

14. *Baggenstoss, A. H.:* The significance of nodular regeneration in cirrhosis of the liver. Am. J. Clin. Path. *25:* 936, 1955.

15. *Baggenstoss, A. H., Soloway, R. D., Summerskill, W. H. J., Elveback, L. R. & Schoenfield, L. J.:* Chronic active liver disease: the range of histologic lesions, their response to treatment, and evolution. Human Path. *3:* 183, 1972.

16. *Bagley, C. M., Roth, J. A., Thomas, L. B. & Devita, V. T.:* Liver biopsy in Hodgkin's disease. Ann intern. Med. *76:* 219, 1972.

17. *Bang, J. & Wanscher, O.:* The histopathology of the liver in infectious mononucleosis complicated by jaundice, investigated by aspiration biopsy. Acta med. scand. *120:* 437, 1945.

18. *Barrett, G. M. & Rickards, A. G.:* Chronic brucellosis. Quart J. Med. *85:* 23, 1953.

19. *Baum, J. K., Bookstein, J. J., Holtz, F. & Klein, E. W.:* Possible association between benign hepatomas and oral contraceptives. Lancet *ii:* 926, 1973.

20. *Baum, S.:* Hepatic angiography. In: Popper, H. & Schaffner, F. (ed.): Progress in Liver Diseases. vol. 3. New York: Grune & Stratton. p. 444, 1970.

21. *Bell, E. T.:* The relation of portal cirrhosis to hemochromatosis and to diabetes mellitus. Diabetes *4:* 435, 1955.

22. *Benacerraf, B.:* Functions of the Kupffer cells. In: Rouiller, C. H. (ed.): The Liver, Morphology, Biochemistry, Physiology, vol. 2. New York: Academic Press. p. 37, 1964.

23. *Bengelsdorf, H. & Elias, H.:* The structure of the liver of Cyclostomata. Chicago Med. Sch. Quart. *12:* 7, 1950.

24. *Bennike, T.:* Liver Studies in Infectious Mononucleosis and some Acute Infectious Diseases with Special Regard to the Occurrence of Chronic Sequelae. Thesis. Copenhagen: Munksgaard, p. 142, 1960.

25. *Beringer, A. & Thaler, H.:* The relationship between diabetes mellitus and fatty liver. Germ. med. Mth. *15:* 615, 1970.

26. *Berlin, S. O. & Brante, G.:* Iron metabolism in porphyria and hemochromatosis. Lancet *ii:* 729, 1962.

27. *Bero, G. L.:* Amyloidosis: Its clinical and pathologic manifestations, with a report of 12 cases. Ann. Intern. Med. *46:* 931, 1957.

28. *Bianchi, L.:* Punktat-Morphologie und Differentialdiagnose der Hepatitis. Bern und Stuttgart: Vorlag Hans Huber, p. 37, 1968.

29. *Bianchi, L., De Groote, J., Desmet, V., Gedigk, P., Korb, G., Popper, H., Poulsen, H., Scheuer, P., Schmid, M., Thaler, H. & Wepler, W.:* Morphological criteria in viral hepatitis. Lancet *i:* 333, 1971.

30. *Bianchi, L., De Groote, J., Desmet, V., Gedigk, P., Korb, G., Popper, H., Poulsen, H., Scheuer, P., Schmid, M., Thaler, H. & Wepler, W.:* Guidelines for the diagnosis of therapeutic drug-induced liver injury in liver biopsies. Lancet *i:* 854, 1974.

31. *Bianchi, L., De Groote, J., Desmet, V., Gedigk, P., Korb, G., Popper, H., Poulsen, H., Scheuer, P., Schmid, M., Thaler, H. & Wepler, W.:* Acute and chronic hepatitis revisited. Lancet *ii:* 914, 1977.

32. *Bianchi, L. & Gudat, F.:* Histologische Characteristika und Nachweis von Hepatitis-B-Antigen-Komponenten in Lebergewebe bei akuter und chronischer Virushepatitis. Immunität und Infektion *3:* 159, 1975.

33. *Bianchi, L. & Gudat, F.:* Sanded nuclei in hepatitis B. Eosinophilic inclusions in liver cell nuclei due to excess in hepatitis B core antigen formation. Lab. Invest. *35:* 1, 1976.

34. *Bianchi, L., Ohnacker, H., Beck, K. & Zimmerli-Ning, M.:* Liver damage in heatstroke and its regression. Human Path. *3,* 237, 1972.

35. *Biava, C. G.:* Studies on cholestasis. A re-evaluation of the fine structure of normal human bile canaliculi. Lab. Invest. *13:* 840, 1964.

36. *Biava, C. & Muklova-Montiel, M.:* Electron microscopic observations on Councilman-like acidophilic bodies and other forms of acidophilic changes in human liver cells. Am. J. Path. *46:* 775, 1965.

37. *Birgens, H. S., Henriksen, J., Matzen, P. & Poulsen, H.:* Shock liver: The clinical and biochemical findings in patients with centrilobular liver necrosis following cardiogenic shock. Acta med. scand. (in press).

38. *Blackwell, J. B. & Joske, R. A.:* Küpffercell sarcoma. Am. J. Dig. Dis. *15:* 133, 1970.

39. *Blan, A. K., Grand, R. J. & Coltan, H. R.:* Liver in alpha-l-antitrypsin deficiency. Morphological observation and in vitro synthesis of alpha-l-antitrypsin. Pediat. Res. *10:* 35, 1976.

40. *Boyer, J. L. & Klatskin, G.:* Pattern of necrosis in acute viral hepatitis. Prognostic value of bridging (subacute hepatic necrosis). N. Engl. J. Med. *283:* 1063, 1970.

41. *Brachet, J.:* La localisation des acides pentosenucliques dans les tissue animaux et les aufs d'Amphibiens en voie de development. Arch. de biol. *53:* 207, 1942.

42. *Bras, G. & Hill, K. R.:* Veno-occlusive disease of the liver. Essential pathology. Lancet *ii:* 161, 1956.

43. *Braunstein, H.:* Needle biopsy of the liver in cirrhosis. Arch. Path. *62:* 87, 1956.

44. *Bronfenmajer, S., Schaffner, F. & Popper, H.:* Fat-storing cells (lipocytes) in human liver. Arch. Path. *82:* 447, 1966.

45. *Brooke, B. N. & Slaney, G.:* Portal bacteremia in ulcerative colitis. Lancet *i:* 1206, 1958.

46. *Brown, R. E. & Ishak, K. G.:* Hepatic zonal degeneration and necrosis in Reye syndrome. Arch. Path. & Lab. Med. *100:* 123, 1976.

47. *Buntine, D. W., Lyall, I. G. & Renowden, V. G.:* Haemangioendothelial sarcoma of the liver. Med. J. Australia *1:* 201, 1971.

48. *Burdette, W. J.:* Neoplasma of the Liver. In: Schiff, L. (ed.): Diseases of the liver. 4th ed. Philadelphia: Lippincott, p. 1051, 1975.

49. *Burkel, W. E. & Low, F. N.:* The fine structure of rat liver sinusoids, space of Disse, and associated tissue space. Am. J. Anat. *118:* 769, 1966.

50. *Burston, J.:* Küppfer-cell sarcoma. Cancer, *2:* 798, 1958.

51. *Carroll, R.:* Infarction of the human liver. J. Clin. Path. *16:* 133, 1963.

52. *Castberg, T.:* Vascular changes in chronic passive congestion of the liver. Acta path. microbiol. scand. *30:* 358, 1952.

53. *Cavalli, G., Bianchi, F. B., Bacci, G. & Casali, A. M.:* The histogenesis and clinical significance of acidophilic bodies in various liver diseases. Digestion. *1:* 353, 1968.

54. *Charlton, R. W., Jacobs, P., Seftel, H. & Bothwell, T. H.:* Effect of alcohol on iron absorption. Brit. med. J. *2:* 1427, 1964.

55. *Christoffersen, P.:* The incidence and frequency of Mallory bodies in 1.100 consecutive liver biopsies. Acta path. microbiol. scand. Section A. *78:* 395, 1970.

56. *Christoffersen, P.:* Light microscopical features in liver biopsies with Mallory bodies. Acta path. microbiol. scand. Section A. *80:* 705, 1972.

57. *Christoffersen, P., Brændstrup, O., Juhl, E. & Poulsen, H.:* Lipogranulomas in human liver biopsies with fatty change. Acta path microbiol. scand. Section A. *79:* 150, 1971.

58. *Christoffersen, P. & Dietrichson, O.:* Histological changes in liver biopsies from patients with chronic hepatitis. Acta path. microbiol. scand. Section A. *82:* 539, 1974.

59. *Christoffersen, P., Dietrichson, O., Faber, V. & Poulsen, H.:* The occurrence and significance of abnormal bile duct epithelium in chronic aggressive hepatitis. Acta path. microbiol. scand. Section A. *80:* 294, 1972.

60. *Christoffersen, P., Eghøje, K. & Juhl, E.:* Mallory bodies in liver biopsies from chronic alcoholics. Scand. J. Gastroent. *8:* 341, 1973.

61. *Christoffersen, P., Iversen, K., Nielsen, K. & Poulsen, H.:* Alcoholic hepatitis. Scand. J. Gastroent. *5:* 633, 1970.

62. *Christoffersen, P. & Juhl, E.:* Mallory bodies in liver biopsies with fatty change but no cirrhosis. Acta path. microbiol. scand. Section A. *79:* 201, 1971.

63. *Christoffersen, P. & Juhl, E.:* The prognostic significance of Mallory bodies in cirrhosis with fatty change. Scand. J. Gastroent. *8:* 225, 1973.

64. *Christoffersen, P. & Juhl, E.:* The significance of Mallory bodies in the progression of fatty liver into cirrhosis. Acta path. microbiol. scand. Section A. *82:* 483, 1974.

65. *Christoffersen, P. & Nielsen, K.:* The frequency of Mallory bodies in liver biopsies from chronic alcoholics. Acta path. microbiol. scand. Section A. *79:* 274, 1971.

66. *Christoffersen, P. & Nielsen, K.:* Histological changes in human liver biopsies from chronic alcoholics. Acta path. microbiol. scand. Section A. *80:* 557, 1972.

67. *Christoffersen, P. & Poulsen, H.:* Histological changes in human liver biopsies following extrahepatic biliary obstruction. Acta path. microbiol. scand. Suppl. *212:* 150, 1970.

68. *Christoffersen, P. & Poulsen, H.:* Alcoholic liver disease. In: MacSween, R. N. M., Anthony, P. P. & Scheuer, P. J. (ed.): Pathology of the Liver. Edinburgh: Churchill Livingstone, (in press).

69. *Christoffersen, P., Poulsen, H. & Scheuer, P.:* Abnormal bile duct epithelium in chronic aggressive hepatitis and primary biliary cirrhosis. Human Path. *3:* 227, 1972.

70. *Christoffersen, P., Poulsen, H. & Skeie, E.:* Focal liver cell necrosis accompanied by infiltration of granulocytes arising during operation. Acta Hepato-Splenologica (Stuttgart) *17:* 240, 1970.

71. *Christoffersen, P., Poulsen, H. & Winkler, K.:* Clinical findings in patients with hepatitis and abnormal bile duct epithelium. Scand. J. Gastroent. *5:* 117, 1970.

72. *Clara, M.:* Untersuchungen an der menschlichen Leber. I. Über den Übergang der Gallenkapillaren in die Gallengänge. Z. Mikr. Anat. Forsch. *20:* 584, 1930.

73. *Clarke, W. T. T.:* Centrilobular hepatic necrosis following cardiac infarction. Am. J. Path. *26:* 249, 1950.

74. *Cohen, A. S. & Calkins, E.:* Electron microscopic observations on a fibrous component in amyloid of diverse origins. Nature, *183:* 1202, 1959.

75. *Cohen, A. S. & Skinner, M.:* Amyloidosis of the Liver. In: Schiff, L. (ed.): Diseases of the Liver. 4th ed. Philadelphia: Lippincott, p. 1017, 1975.

76. *Cohen, S., Kaplan, M., Gottlieb, L. & Patterson, J.:* Liver disease and gallstones in regional enteritis. Gastroenterology *60:* 237, 1971.

77. *Conn, H. O.:* Chronic hepatitis: reducing an iatrogenic enigma to a workable puzzle. Gastroenterology *70:* 1182, 1976.

78. *Conney, A. H.:* Pharmacytological implications of microsomal enzyme induction. Pharmalogical Reviews *19:* 317, 1967.

79. *Cook, G. C. & Hutt, M. S. R.:* The liver after kwashiorkor. Brit. Med. J. *ii:* 454, 1967.

80. *Cossel, L.:* Über den submikroskopishen Zusammenhang der interzellulären Räume und Sinusoide in der Leber. Z. Zellforsch. *58:* 76, 1960.

81. *Cossel, L.:* Beitrag zur submikroschopischen Morphologie des Stoffaustausches und intrazellulären Stofftransportes in der Leber. Acta Hepatosplen. (Stuttgart) *8:* 264, 1961.

82. *Cossel, L.:* Elektronmikroskopische Befunde am Übergang der intralobulären Gallen-Kanälchen in die Gallengänge. Virchow Arch. Path. Anat. *335:* 647, 1962.

83. *Cripps, D. J. & Scheuer, P. J.:* Hepatobiliary changes in erythropoietic protoporphyria. Arch. Path. *80:* 500, 1965.

84. *Cruickshank, A. H.:* The pathology of 111 cases of primary hepatic malignancy collected in the Liverpool region. J. Clin. Path. *14:* 120, 1961.

85. *Da Silva, J. R. & De Paola, D.:* Hepatic lesions in American kala-azar: a needle biopsy study. Ann. trop. Med. Parasit. *55:* 249, 1961.

86. *Datta, D. V., Saha, S., Samanta, A. K. S., Gupta, B. B., Aikat, B. K., Chugh, K. S. & Chuttani, P. N.:* Chronic Budd-Chiari syndrome due to obstruction of the intrahepatic portion of the inferior vena cava. GUT. *13:* 372, 1972.

87. *David-Ferreira, J. F. & David-Ferreira, K. L.:* Gap junction – ribosome association after autolysis. J. Cell. Biol. *58:* 226, 1973.

88. *Davies, J. N. P.:* Hepatic neoplasm. In: Gall, E. A. & Mostofi, F. K. (ed.): The Liver. International Academy of Pathology. Monographs 13. Baltimore: Williams & Wilkins, p. 361, 1973.

89. *De Groote, J., Desmet, V., Gedigk, P., Korb, G., Popper, H., Poulsen, H., Scheuer, P. J., Schmid, M., Thaler, H., Uehlinger, E. & Wepler, W.:* A classification of chronic hepatitis. Lancet, *ii:* 626, 1968.

90. *Dehner, L. P. & Ishak, K. G.:* Vascular tumors of the liver in infants and children. A study of 30 cases and review of the literature. Arch. Path. *92:* 101, 1971.

91. *De Man, J. C. H. & Blok, A. P. R.:* Relationship between glycogen and agranular endoplasmic reticulum in rat hepatic cells. J. Histochem. Cytochem. *14:* 135, 1966.

92. *Desmet, V. J.:* Morphologic and histochemical aspects of cholestasis. In: Popper, H. & Schaffner, F. (ed.): Progress in Liver Diseases. Vol. 4. New York: Grune & Stratton, p. 97, 1972.

93. *Desmet, V. J.:* Chronic hepatitis (including primary biliary cirrhosis). In: Gall, E. A. & Mostofi, F. K. (ed.): The Liver. International Academy of Pathology. Monographs. 13, Baltimore: Williams & Wilkins, p. 286, 1973.

94. *Desmet, V. J.:* Morphogenesis of chronic hepatitis. Europ. Med. (in Press).

95. *Desmet, V. J., Bullens, A. M. & De Groote, J.:* A clinical and histochemical study of cholestases. GUT. *11:* 516, 1970.

96. *Desmet, V. J. & De Groote, J.:* Histological diagnosis of viral hepatitis. In: Tygstrup, N. (ed.): Viral Hepatitis. Clinics in Gastroenterology. Vol. 3. London: Saunders. 337, 1974.

97. *Desmet, V. J., De Groote, J. & Van Damme, B.:* Acute hepatocellular failure. Human Path. *3:* 167, 1972.

98. *Dietrichson, O.:* Chronic persistent hepatitis. A clinical, serological and prognostic study. Scand. J. Gastroent. *10:* 249, 1975.

99. *Dietrichson, O. & Christoffersen, P.:* The prognosis of chronic aggressive hepatitis. Scand. J. Gastroent. *12:* 289, 1977.

100. *Dietrichson, O., From, A., Christoffersen, P. & Juhl, E.:* Morphological changes in liver biopsies from patients with rheumatoid arthritis. Scand. J. Rheum. *5:* 65, 1976.

101. *Dietrichson, O., Juhl, E., Christoffersen, P., Elling, P., Faber, V., Iversen, K., Nielsen, J. O., Petersen, P. & Poulsen, H.:* Acute viral hepatitis: Factors possibly predicting chronic liver disease. Acta path. microbiol. scand. Section A: *83:* 183, 1975.

102. *Di Luzio, N. R.:* Prevention of the acute ethanol-induced fatty liver by simultaneous administration of antioxidants. Life Sciences *3:* 113, 1964.

103. *Doehlert, C. A. J., Baggenstoss, A. H. & Cain, J. C.:* Obstructive biliary cirrhosis and alcoholic cirrhosis: Comparison of clinical and pathologic features. Am. J. Clin. Path. *25:* 902, 1955.

104. *Doniach, D. & Walker, J. G.:* A unified concept of autoimmune hepatitis. Lancet *i:* 813, 1969.

105. *Dordal, E., Glagov, S., Orlando, R. A. & Platz, C.:* Fatal halothane hepatitis with transient granulomas. N. Engl. J. Med. *283:* 357, 1970.

106. *Dordal, E., Glagov, S. & Kirsner, J. B.:* Hepatic lesions in chronic inflammatory bowel disease. I. Clinical correlations with liver biopsy diagnosis in 103 patients. Gastroenterology *52:* 239, 1967.

107. *Dubin, I. N.:* Chronic idiopathic jaundice. Am. J. Med. *24:* 268, 1958.

108. *Du Bois, A. M.:* The embryonic liver. In: Rouiller, C. (ed.): The Liver: Morphology, Biochemistry, Physiology. Vol. 1. New York: Academic Press, p. 1, 1963.

109. *Eade, M. N.:* Liver disease in ulcerative colitis. I. Analysis of operative liver biopsy in 138 consecutive patients having colectomy. Ann. Int. Med. *72:* 475, 1970.

110. *Edington, G. M.:* Pathology of malaria in West Africa. Brit. med. J. *i:* 715, 1967.

111. *Edmondson, H. A.:* Tumours of the liver and intrahepatic bile ducts. In: Atlas of Tumor Pathology. Washington D. C.: A. F. I. P. Section VII, pp. 32[a], 49[b], 80[c], 216[d], 1958.

112. *Edmondson, H. A., Hendersen, B. & Benton, B.:* Liver-cell adenomas associated with use of oral contraceptives. N. Eng. J. Med. *294:* 470, 1976.

113. *Edmondson, H. A., Peters, R. L., Reynolds, T. B. & Kuzma, O. T.:* Sclerosing hyalin necrosis of the liver in chronic alcoholics: A recognizable clinical syndrome. Ann. Int. Med. *59:* 646, 1963.

114. *Edmondson, H. A. & Steiner, P. E.:* Primary carcinoma of the liver; a study of 100 cases among 48.900 necropsies. Cancer *7:* 462, 1954.

115. *Edwards, G. A. & Zawadski, Z. A.:* Extraosseous lesions in plasma cell myeloma. Am. J. Med. *43:* 194, 1967.

116. *Ekman, C. A. & Holmgren, H.:* The effect of alimentary factors on liver glycogen rhythm and the distribution of glycogen in the liver lobule. Anat. Rec. *104:* 189, 1949.

117. *El-Domeiri, A. A., Huros, A. G., Goldsmith, H. E. & Foote, F. W.:* Primary malignant tumors of the liver. Cancer *27:* 7, 1971.

118. *Elias, H.:* The liver cord concept after one hundred years. Science *110:* 470, 1949.

119. *Elias, H.:* A re-examination of the structure of the mammalian liver. I. Parenchymal architecture. Am. J. Anat. *84:* 311, 1949.

120. *Elias, H.:* A re-examination of the structure of the mammalian liver. II. The hepatic lobule and its relation to the vascular and biliary system. Am. J. Anat. *85:* 379, 1949.

121. *Elias, H. & Petty, D.:* Gross anatomy of the blood vessels and ducts within the human liver. Am. J. Anat. *90:* 59, 1952.

122. *Elias, H. & Popper, H.:* Venous distribution in livers; comparison of man and experimental animals and application to morphogenesis of cirrhosis. Arch. Path. *59:* 332, 1955.

123. *Elias, H. & Popper, H.:* Histodynamik der Leberzirrhose. Acta Hepatosplen. (Stuttgart) *4:* 2, 1956.

124. *Elias, H. & Sherrick, J. C.:* Morphology of the liver. New York & London: Academic Press, p. 13, 1969.

125. *Elias, H. & Sokol, A.:* Dependence of the lobular architecture of the liver on the porto-hepatic blood pressure gradient. Anat. Rec. *115:* 71, 1953.

126. *Eriksson, S. & Larsson, C.:* Purification and partial characterization of PAS-positive inclusion bodies from the liver in alpha-l-antitrypsin deficiency. N. Engl. J. Med. *292:* 176, 1975.

127. *Espiritu, C. R., Kim, T. S. & Levine, R. A.:* Granulomatous hepatitis associated with sulfadimethoxine hypersensitivity. J. A. M. A. *202:* 985, 1967.

128. *Essner, E. & Novikoff, A. B.:* Human hepatocellular pigments and lysosomes. J. Ultrastruct. Res. *3:* 374, 1960.

129. *Farber, E.:* Environmental factors in the development of liver cancer. In: Schaffner, F., Sherlock, S. & Leevy, C. M. (ed.): The Liver and Its Diseases. Stuttgart: Thieme, p. 337, 1974.

130. *Fawcett, D. W.:* Observations on the cytology and electron microscopy of hepatic cells. J. Nat. Cancer Inst. *15:* 1475, 1955.

131. *Finckh, E. S., Baker, S. F. & Ryam, M. M. P.:* The value of liver biopsy in the diagnosis of tuberculosis and sarcoidosis. Med. J. Aus. *2:* 369, 1953.

132. *Fischer, R., Taylor, L., Maze, M. & Sherlock, S.:* α-l-antitrypsin deficiency in liver disease: The extent of the problem. Digestion *10:* 320, 1974.

133. *Frederickson, D. S. & Sloan, H. R.:* Glucosyl ceramide lipidoses (Gaucher's disease). In: Stanbury, J. B. (ed.): The Metabolic Basis of Inherited Disease. 3rd. ed. New York: Mc Graw Hill, p. 730, 1972.

134. *Frommer. J.:* The pathogenesis of reticuloendothelial foam cells; effect of polyvinylpyrrolidone on the liver of the mouse. Am. J. Path. *32:* 433, 1956.

135. *Gall, E. A., Williams, A., Altemeier, A., Schiff, L., Hamilton, D. L., Braunstein, H., Guiseffi, J. & Freimann, D. G.:* Liver lesions following intraveneous administration of polyvinyl pyrrolidone (PVP). Am. J. Clin. Path. *23:* 1187, 1953.

136. *Gall, E. A.:* Primary and metastatic carcinoma of the liver – relationship to hepatic cirrhosis. Arch. Path. *70:* 226, 1960.

137. *Gall, E. A.:* Posthepatic, postnecrotic and nutritional cirrhosis. Am. J. Path. *36:* 241, 1960.

138. *Gall, E. A. & Dobrogorski, O.:* Hepatic alterations in obstructive jaundice. Am. J. Clin. Path. *41:* 126, 1964.

139. *Gall, E. A. & Landing, B. H.:* Hepatic cirrhosis and hereditary disorders of metabolism. Am. J. Path. *26:* 1398, 1956.

140. *Geddes, E. W. & Falkson, G.:* Malignant hepatoma in the Bantu. Cancer *25:* 1271, 1970.

141. *Gentz, J., Jagenburg, R. & Zetterstrøm, R.:* Tyrosinemia. J. Pediat. *66:* 670, 1965.

142. *Gerber, M. A., Orr, W., Denk, H., Schaffner, F. & Popper, H.:* Hepatocellular hyaline in cholestasis and cirrhosis: its diagnostic significance. Gastroenterology *64:* 89, 1973.

143. *Gerber, M. A. & Popper, H.:* Relation between central canals and portal tracts in alcoholic hepatitis. A contribution to the pathogenesis of cirrhosis in alcoholics. Hum. Path. *3:* 199, 1972.

144. *Gerber, M. A. & Vernace, S.:* Chronic septal hepatitis. Virchows Arch. *363:* 303, 1974.

145. *Givler, R. L., Brunk, S. F., Hass, C. A. & Gulesserian, H. P.:* Problems of interpretation of liver biopsy in Hodgkins disease. Cancer *28:* 1335, 1971.

146. *Goldstein, G.:* Sarcoid reaction associated with phenylbutazone hypersensitivity. Ann. intern. med. *59:* 97, 1963.

147. *Grace, N. D. & Powell, L. W.:* Iron storage disorders of the liver. Gastroenterology *64:* 1257, 1974.

148. *Greiner, A. C. & Nicolson, G. A.:* Pigment deposition in viscera associated with prolonged chlorpromazine therapy. Can. med. Ass. J. *91:* 627, 1964.

149. *Gubetta, L., Rizzetto, M., Crivelli, O., Verme, G. & Arico, S.:* A trichrome stain for the intrahepatic localization of the hepatitis B surface antigen (HB$_S$Ag). Histopathology *1:* 277, 1977.

150. *Guckian, J. C. & Perry, J. E.:* Granulomatous hepatitis. Ann. intern. Med. *65:* 1081, 1966.

151. *Gudat, F., Bianchi, L., Sonnabend, W., Thiel, G., Aenishaenslin, W. & Stalder, G. A.:* Pattern of core and surface expression in liver tissue reflects state of specific immune response in hepatitis B. Lab. Invest. *32:* 1, 1975.

152. *Hadziyannis, S., Gerber, M. A., Vissoulis, C. Y. & Popper, H.:* Cytoplasmic hepatitis B antigen in "ground-glass" hepatocytes of carriers. Arch. Path. *96:* 327, 1973.

153. *Hadziyannis, S., Scheuer, P. J., Feizi, T., Naccarato, R., Doniach, D. & Sherlock, S.:* Immunological and histological studies in primary biliary cirrhosis. J. Clin. Path. *23:* 95, 1970.

154. *Hanshaw, J. B., Betts, R. F., Simon, G. & Boynton, R. C.:* Acquired cytomegalovirus infection. N. Engl. J. Med. *272:* 602, 1965.

155. *Harris, R. C., Andersen, D. H. & Day, R. L.:* Obstructive jaundice in infants with normal biliary tree. Pediatrics *13:* 293, 1954.

156. *Healey, J. E. & Schroy, P. C.:* The anatomy of the bile ducts within the human liver: An analysis of the prevailing patterns of branching and their major variants. Arch. Surg. *66:* 599, 1953.

157. *Higginson, J.:* The geographic pathology of primary liver cancer. Cancer Res. *23:* 1624, 1963.

158. *Hilden, M, Juhl, E., Thomsen, Å. Chr. & Christoffersen, P.:* Fatty liver persisting for up to 33 years. Acta med scand. *194:* 485, 1973.

159. *Hirooka, M. & Kimura, C.:* Membraneous obstruction of the hepatic portion of the inferior vena cava. Arch. Surg. *100:* 656, 1970.

160. *Hjortsö, C. H.:* The topography of the intrahepatic duct system. Acta Anat. *11:* 599, 1951.

161. *Horta, J. Das.:* Late effects of thorotrast on the liver and spleen, and their efferent lymphnodes. Ann. N. Y. Acad. Sci. *145:* 676, 1967.

162. *Hunt, A. H., Parr, R. M., Taylor, D. M. & Trott, N. G.:* Relationship between cirrhosis and trace metal content of liver. Brit. med. J. *ii:* 1498, 1963.

163. *Hunter, F. M., Akdamar, K., Sparks, R. D., Reed, R. J. & Brown, C. L.:* Congenital dilatation of the intrahepatic bile ducts. Am. J. Med. *40:* 188, 1966.

164. *Hutterer, F., Eisenstadt, M. & Rubin, E.:* Turnover of hepatic collagen in reversible and irreversible hepatic fibrosis. Experientia *26:* 244, 1970.

165. *Iseri, O. A. & Gottlieb, L. S.:* "Alcoholic hyaline" and enlarged mitochondria as distinct entities in alcoholic liver disease. Fed. Proc. *27:* 605, 1968.

166. *Ishak, K. G.:* Viral hepatitis. The morphologic spectrum. In: Gall, F. A. & Mostofi, F. K. (ed.): The Liver. International Academy of Pathology. Monographs 13. Baltimore: Williams & Wilkins, p. 218, 1973.

167. *Ishak, K. G., Jenis, E. H., Marshall, M. L., Bolton, B. H. & Baltistone, G. C.:* Cirrhosis of the liver associated with alpha-1-antitrypsin deficiency. Arch. Path. *94:* 445, 1972.

168. *Israel, H. L. & Sones, M.:* Selection of biopsy procedures for sarcoidosis diagnosis. Arch. intern. Med. *113:* 255, 1964.

169. *Ito, T. & Nemoto, M.:* Über die Kupfferschen Sternzellen und die „Fettspeicherungzellen" („fat-storing cells") in der Blutkapillarenwand der menschlichen Leber. Okajima Folia Anat. Jap. *24:* 243, 1952.

170. *Iversen, K., Christoffersen, P. & Poulsen, H.:* Epitheioid cell granulomas in liver biopsies. Scand. J. Gastroent. Suppl. *7:* 61, 1970.

171. *Javitt, N. B.:* Neonatal cholestatic syndromes. A structure-function dilemma. Viewpoints on Digestive Diseases *5:* 1, 1973.

172. *Jones, J. M. & Peck, W. M.:* Incidence of fatty liver in tuberculosis with special reference to tuberculous enteritis. Arch. Int. Med. *74:* 371, 1944.

173. *Jørgensen, M.:* A case of abnormal intrahepatic bile duct arrangement submitted to three dimensional reconstruction. Acta path. microbiol. scand. Section A. *79:* 303, 1971.

174. *Kaman, J.:* Zur terminalen Ramifikation der Arteria hepatica des Schweines. Mikroskopie *20:* 129, 1965.

175. *Karmi, G., Thirkettle, J. L. & Read, A. E. A.:* The association of syphilis with hepatic cirrhosis: A report of six cases and a review of the literature. Postgrad med. J. *45:* 675, 1969.

176. *Karvountzis, G., Redeker, A. G. & Peters, R. L.:* Long term follow-up studies of patients surviving fulminal viral hepatitis. Gastroenterology *67:* 870, 1974.

177. *Kay, S. & Schatzki, P. F.:* Ultrastructure of a benign liver cell adenoma. Cancer *28:* 755, 1971.

178. *Keller, T. C. & Smetana, H. F.:* Artefacts in liver biopsies. Am. J. Clin. Path. *20:* 738, 1950.

179. *Kent, G. & Popper, H.:* Secondary hemochromatosis: Its association with anemia. Arch. Path. *70:* 623, 1960.

180. *Kent, G. & Popper, H.:* Liver biopsy in diagnosis of hemochromatosis. Am. J. Med. *44:* 837, 1968.

181. *Kent, G., Gay, S., Inouye, T., Bahu, R., Minick, O. T. & Popper, H.:* Vitamin A-containing lipocytes and formation of type III collagen in liver injury. Proc. Natl. Acad. Sci U. S. A. *73:* 3719, 1976.

182. *Kent, G. & Schneider, K. A.:* Cirrhosis and iron overload. In: Schaffner, F., Sherlock, S. & Leevy, C. M. (ed.): The Liver and Its Diseases. Stuttgart: Thieme, p. 314, 1974.

183. *Kerr, D. N. S., Harrison, C. V., Sherlock, S. & Milnes Walker, R.:* Congenital hepatic fibrosis. Quart. J. Med. *30:* 91, 1961.

184. *Kerr, J. F. R.:* Shrinkage necrosis. A distinct mode of cellular death. J. Path. *105:* 13, 1971.

185. *Khilnani, M. T.:* Calcified liver metastasis from carcinoma of the colon. Am. J. Dig. Dis. *6:* 229, 1961.

186. *Kirschbaum, J. D. & Preuss, F. S.:* Leukemia. A clinical and pathologic study of 123 fatal cases in a series of 14.400 necropsies. Arch. Int. Med. *71:* 777, 1943.

187. *Klatskin, G.:* Toxic and drug-induced hepatitis. In: Schiff, L. (ed.): Diseases of the Liver. 4th ed. Philadelphia: Lippincott, p. 604, 1975.

188. *Klatskin, G.:* Hepatitis associated with systemic infections. In: Schiff, L. (ed.): Diseases of the Liver. 4th. ed. Philadelphia: Lippincott, p. 711, 1975.

189. *Klatskin, G.:* Hepatic tumours. Possible relationship to use of oral contraceptives. Gastroenterology *73:* 386, 1977.

190. *Klatskin, G. & Yesner, R.:* Hepatic manifestations of sarcoidosis and other granulomatous diseases: A study based on histological examination of tissue obtained by needle biopsy of the liver. Yale J. Biol. Med. *23:* 207, 1950.

191. *Klion, F. M. & Schaffner, F.:* The ultrastructure of acidophilic "Councilman-like" bodies in the liver. Am. J. Path. *48:* 755, 1966.

192. *Klion, F. M., Schaffner, F. & Popper, H.:* Hepatitis after exposure to halothane. Ann. Intern. Med. *71:* 467, 1969.

193. *Knisely, M. H., Bloch, E. H. & Warner, L.:* Selective phagocytosis I. Microscopic observations concerning the regulation of the blood flow through the liver and other organs and the mechanism and rate of phagocytic removal of particles from the blood. Kgl. Danske Videnskab. Selskab. Biol. Skrifter *4:* 1, 1948.

194. *Korb, G., Mohren, W. & Weiss, R.:* Chirurgische granulozytäre Leberzellnekrosen und Bedeutung intraoperativer Leberbiopsien. Leber Magen Darm. *7:* 277, 1977.

195. *Kunelis, C. T., Peters, J. L. & Edmondson, H. A.:* Fatty liver of pregnancy and its relationship to tetracycline therapy. Am. J. Med. *38:* 359, 1965.

196. *Kwittken, J. & Tartow, L. R.:* Haemochromatosis and Küpffercell sarcoma with unusual localization of iron. J. Path. Bact. *92:* 571, 1966.

197. *Leduc, E. H. & Wilson, J. W.:* An electron microscope study of intranuclear inclusions in mouse liver and hepatoma. J. biophys. biochem. Cytol. *6:* 427, 1959.

198. *Lee, R. V., Thornton, G. F. & Conn, H. O.:* Liver disease associated with secondary syphilis. N. Engl. J. Med. *284:* 1423, 1971.

199. *Leopold, J. G., Parry, T. E. & Storring, F. K.:* A change in the sinusoid-trabecular structure of the liver with hepatic venous outflow block. J. Path. *100:* 87, 1970.

200. *Levi, A. J., Sherlock, S., Scheuer, P. J. & Cumings, J. N.:* Presymptomatic Wilson's disease. Lancet *ii:* 575, 1967.

201. *Levin, B., Snodgrass, G. J. A. I., Oberholzer, V. G., Burgess, E. A. & Dobbs, R. H.:* Fructosaemia. Am. J. Med. *45:* 826, 1968.

202. *Levine, R. A.:* Amyloid disease of the liver: Correlation of clinical, functional and morphologic features in 47 patients. Am. J. Med. *33:* 349, 1962.

203. *Lieber, C. S.:* Alcohol and the liver. In: Popper, H. Schaffner, F. (ed.): Progress in Liver Diseases. Vol. 2. New York: Grune & Stratton, p. 134, 1965.

204. *Lieberman, J., Mittmann, C. & Gordon, H. W.:* Alpha-l-antitrypsin in the livers of patients with emphysema. Science *175:* 63, 1972.

205. *Lindquist, R. R.:* Studies on the pathogenesis of hepatolenticular degeneration. II. Cytochemical methods for the localization of copper. Arch. Path. *87:* 370, 1969.

206. *Lison, L. & Dagnelie, J.:* Methods nouvelles de coloration de la Myéline. Bull. Histol. appl. *12:* 85, 1935.

207. *Lucke, V. & Mallory, T.:* The fulminant form of epidemic hepatitis. Am. J. Path. *22:* 867, 1946.

208. *Ludwig, J.:* A review of lobular, portal, and periportal hepatitis. Interpretation of biopsy specimens without clinical data. Human Path. *8:* 269, 1977.

209. *Lundvall, O. & Enerbäck, L.:* Hepatic fluorescense in porphyria cutanea tarda studied in fine needle aspiration biopsy smears. J. Clin. Path. *22:* 704, 1969.

210. *Lyon, H. & Becher Carstens, P. H.:* Light microscopic studies on the distribution of glycogen in human liver biopsies with special reference to the limiting plate. Acta path. microbiol. scand. *71:* 502, 1967.

211. *Lyon, H. & Christoffersen, P.:* Histochemical study of Mallory bodies. Acta path. microbiol. scand. Section A. *79:* 649, 1971.

212. *Lyon, H. & Prentø, P.:* Artefactual staining of the peripheral zone of needle biopsies. Acta path. microbiol. scand. Section A. *81:* 9, 1973.

213. *Ma, M. H. & Biempica, L.:* The normal human liver cell. Cytochemical and ultrastructural studies. Am. J. Path. *62:* 353, 1971.

214. *MacMahon, H. E.:* Über die physiologische und pathologische Teilung von Kern und Zelle an Leber-epithelien. Z. Mikr. Anat. Forsch. *32:* 413, 1933.

215. *Macleod, M. & Stalker, A. L.:* Diagnosis of Hodgkins disease by liver biopsy. Brit. Med. J. *i:* 1449, 1962.

216. *Maddrey, W. C., Johns, C. J., Boitnott, J. K. & Iber, F. L.:* Sarcoidosis and chronic hepatic disease: A clinical and pathological study of 20 patients. Medicine *49:* 375, 1970.

217. *Mahadevan, S. & Tappel, A. L.:* Lysosomal lipases of rat liver and kidney. J. Biol. Chem. *243:* 2849, 1968.

218. *Mahler, R.:* Glycogen storage diseases. J. Clin. Path. *22 suppl. 2:* 32, 1969.

219. *Majno, G., La Guattata, M. & Thomson, T. E.:* Cellular death and necrosis: Chemical, physical and morphological changes in rat liver. Virchows Arch. Path. Anat. *333:* 421, 1960.

220. *Mall, F. P.:* A study of the structural unit of the liver. Am. J. Anat. *5:* 227, 1906.

221. *Mallory, F. B.:* Cirrhosis of the liver. Five different types of lesions from which it may arise. Bull. John Hopkins Hospital *22:* 69, 1911.

222. *Manitz, G. & Themann, H.:* Elektronenmikrosko-pisher Beitrag zur Feinstruktur menschlichen leber-amyloids. Beitr. Path. Anat. U. Z. allg. Path. *128:* 103, 1962.

223. *Markowitz, J. & Rappaport, A. M.:* The hepatic artery. Physiol. Rew. *31:* 188, 1951.

224. *Martin, N. D.:* Macroglobulinaemia. Quart. J. Med. *29:* 179, 1960.

225. *Masuko, K., Rubin, E. & Popper, H.:* Proliferation of bile ducts in cirrhosis. Arch. Path. *78:* 421, 1964.

226. *McAdams, A. J. & Wilson, H. E.:* The liver in generalized glycogen storage disease. Am. J. Path. *49:* 99, 1966.

277. *McCuskey, R. S.:* A dynamic and static study of hepatic arterioles and hepatic sphincters. Am. J. Anat. *119:* 455, 1966.

228. *McFadzean, A. J. S. & Young, W. T.:* Further observations on hypoglycemia in hepatocellular carcinoma. Am. J. Med. *47:* 220, 1969.

229. *McGee, J. O. & Patrick, R. S.:* The role of peri-sinusoidal cells in hepatic fibrogenesis: An electron microscopic study of acute carbon tetrachloride liver injury. Lab. Invest. *26:* 429, 1972.

230. *McMahon, H. E. & Ball, H. G.:* Leiomyosarcoma of hepatic vein and the Budd-Chiari syndrome. Gastroenterology *61:* 239, 1971.

231. *Meldolesc. J.:* On the significance of the hyper-trophy of the smooth endoplasmic reticulum in liver cells after administration of drugs. Biochemical Pharmacology. *16:* 125, 1967.

232. *Melnick, P. J.:* Polycystic liver. Arch. Path. *59:* 162, 1955.

233. *Mikkelsen, W. P., Edmondson, H. A., Peters, R. L., Redeker, A. G. & Reynolds, T. B.:* Extra- and intrahepatic portal hypertension without cirrhosis (hepatoportal sclerosis). Ann. Surg. *162:* 602, 1965.

234. *Miller, D. J., Dwyer, J. M. & Klatskin, G.:* Identi-fication of lymphocytes in percutaneous liver biopsy cores. Different T: B cell ratio in HB_SAg – positive and – negative hepatitis. Gastroenterology *72:* 1199, 1977.

235. *Miller, E. J. & Matakus, V. J.:* Biosynthesis of collagen: The biochemist's view. Fed. Proc. *33:* 1197, 1974.

236. *Miller, J., Mitchell, C. G., Eddleston, A. L. W. F., Smith, M. G. M., Reed, W. D. & Williams, R.:* Cell-mediated immunity to a human liver specific antigen in patients with active chronic hepatitis and primary biliary cirrhosis. Lancet *ii:* 296, 1972.

237. *Minot, C. S.:* On a hitherto unrecognized form of blood circulation without capillaries in the organs of the vertebrata. Proc. Boston. Soc. Natural Hist. *29:* 185, 1900.

238. *Missmahl, H. P. & Hartwig, M.:* Polarisations-optische untersuchungen and der amyloid-substanz. Virchow Arch. Path. Anat. u. Physiol. *324:* 489, 1953.

239. *Mistilis, S. P.:* Chronic active hepatitis. In: Schiff, L. (ed.): Diseases of the Liver. 4th ed. Philadelphia: Lippincott, p. 787, 1975.

240. *Mistilis, S. P. & Blackburn, C. R. B.:* Active chronic hepatitis. Am. J. Med. *48:* 484, 1970.

241. *Morgan, J. D. & Hartroft, W. S.:* Juvenile liver age at which one cell thick plates predominate in the human liver. Arch. Path. *71:* 86, 1961.

242. *Morgan, M. Y., Sherlock, S. & Scheuer, P. J.:* Acute cholestasis, hepatic failure, and fatty liver in the alcoholic. Scand. J. Gastroent. *13:* 299, 1978.

243. *Mori, W.:* Cirrhosis and primary carcinoma of the liver; comparative study in Tokyo and Cincinnati. Cancer *20:* 627, 1967.

244. *Morris, J. S., Schmid, M., Newmann, S., Scheuer, P. J. & Sherlock, S.:* Arsenic and non-cirrhotic portal hypertension. Gastroenterology *66:* 86, 1974.

245. *Mosley, J. W. & Galambos, J.:* Viral hepatitis. In: Schiff, L. (ed.): Diseases of the Liver. 4th ed. Philadelphia: Lippincott, p. 500, 1975.

246. *Motta, P. & Porter, K. R.:* Structure of rat liver sinusoids and associated tissue spaces as revealed by scanning electron microscopy. Cell Tissue Res. *148:* 111, 1974.

247. *Nayak, N. C. & Ramalingaswami, V.:* Obliterative portal venopathy of the liver. Arch. Path. *87:* 359, 1969.

248. *Nelson, R. S. & Salvador, D. S. J.:* Percutaneous needle liver biopsy in malignant neoplasm with special reference to myeloid metaplasia. Ann. Int. Med. *53:* 179, 1960.

249. *Norman, M. G., Lowden, J. A., Hill, D. E. & Bannatyne, R. M.:* Encephalopathy and fatty degeneration of the viscera in childhood: II. Report of a case with isolation of influenza B virus. Canad. med. Ass. J. *99:* 549, 1968.

250. *Nyfors, A. & Poulsen, H.:* Liver biopsies from psoriatics related to methotrexate therapy. Acta path. microbiol. scand. Section A. *84:* 253, 1976.

251. *Page, A. R. & Good, R. A.:* Plasma cell hepatitis. Lab. Invest. *11:* 351, 1962.

252. *Palmer, P. E., Gheradi, G. J., Balduim, I. M. & Wolfe, H. J.:* Adult liver disease in SZ-phenotype alpha-l-antitrypsin deficiency. Ann. Intern. Med. *88:* 59, 1978.

253. *Parets, A. D.:* Detection of intrahepatic metastases by blind needle liver biopsy. Am. J. Med. Sci. *237:* 335, 1959.

254. *Parker, J. C., Dahlin, D. C. & Stauffer, M. H.:* Malignant hepatoma: evaluation of surgical (including needle biopsy) material from 69 cases. Mayo Clinic Proc. *45:* 25, 1970.

255. *Parker, R. G. F.:* Occlusion of the hepatic veins in man. Medicine *38:* 369, 1959.

256. *Paronetto, F. & Popper, H.:* Chronic liver injury induced by immunologic reactions, cirrhosis following immunization with heterologous sera. Am. J. Path. *47:* 549, 1965.

257. *Pearson, A. J. G., Grainger, J. H., Scheuer, P. J. & McIntyre, N.:* Jaundice due to oxyphenisatin. Lancet *i:* 994, 1971.

258. *Perez, V., Royer, M., Garay, E. & Lozzio, B.:* Some electron microscopic features of experimental biliary obstruction. In: Martini, G. (ed.): Aktuelle Probleme der Hepatologie. Stuttgart: Georg Thieme Verlag, p. 47, 1962.

259. *Perez, V., Schaffner, F. & Popper, H.:* Hepatic drug reaction. In: Popper, H. & Schaffner, F. (ed.): Progress in Liver Diseases, Vol. 4. New York: Grune & Stratton, p. 597, 1972.

260. *Perls, M.:* Nachweiss von eisenoxyd in gewissen Pigmenten. Arch. Pathol. Anat. Phys. *39:* 42, 1867.

261. *Peters, R. L., Edmondson, H. A., Mikkelsen, W. P. & Tatter, D.:* Tetracycline induced fatty liver in non-pregnant patients. Am. J. Surg. *113:* 622, 1967.

262. *Peters, R. L., Edmondson, H. A., Reynolds, T. B., Meister, J. C. & Curphey, T. J.:* Hepatic necrosis associated with halothane anesthesia. Am. J. Med. *47:* 748, 1969.

263. *Peters, R. L. & Reynolds, T. B.:* Hepatic changes simulating alcoholic liver disease, post ileojejunal bypass. Gastroenterology *65:* 564, 1973.

264. *Petersen, P. & Christoffersen, P.:* Ultrastructure of lipogranulomas in human fatty liver. Acta path. et microbiologica scand. Section A. (in press).

265. *Petersen, P., Christoffersen, P., Elling, P., Juhl, E., Dietrichson, O., Faber, V., Iversen, K., Nielsen, J. O. & Poulsen, H.:* Acute viral hepatitis A survey of 500 patients. Scand. J. Gastroent. *9:* 607, 1974.

266. *Petrelli, M. & Scheuer, P. J.:* Variation in subcapsular liver structure and its significance in the interpretation of wedge biopsies. J. Clin. Path. *20:* 743, 1967.

267. *Philips, M. J. & Steiner, J. W.:* Electron microscopy of cirrhotic nodules; tubularization of the parenchyma by biliary hepatocytes. Lab. Invest. *15:* 801, 1966.

268. *Platzer, S., Auhuber, I., Geir, W. & Judmaier, G.:* Prognose der akuten virushepatitis B. Leber Magen Darm. *8:* 83, 1978.

269. *Popper, H.:* Significance of agonal changes in human liver. Arch. Path. *46:* 132, 1948.

270. *Popper, H.:* The problem of hepatitis. Am. J. Gastroent. *55:* 335, 1971.

271. *Popper, H.:* The pathology of viral hepatitis. Can. Med. Ass. J. *106:* 447, 1972.

272. *Popper, H.:* Drug-induced liver injury. In: Gall, E. A. & Mostofi, F. K. (ed.): The Liver. International Academy of Pathology. Monographs 13. Baltimore: Williams & Wilkins, p. 182, 1973.

273. *Popper, H.:* Morphologic features of hepatocellular necrosis in human disease. In: Keppler, E. (ed.): Pathogenesis and mechanisms of liver cell necrosis. Lancaster: MTP Press. Ltd., p. 15, 1975.

274. *Popper, H.:* Pathologic aspects of cirrhosis. A review. Am. J. Path. *87:* 228, 1977.

275. *Popper, H. & Kent, G.:* Fibrosis in chronic liver disease. In: Popper, H. (ed.): Clinics in Gastroenterology *4:* Philadelphia: Saunders. p. 315, 1975.

276. *Popper, H. & Orr, W.:* Current concepts in cirrhosis. Scand. J. Gastroent. *6:* 203, 1970.

277. *Popper, H., Paronetto, F. & Barka, T.:* PAS-positive structures of nonglycogenic character in normal and abnormal liver. Arch. Path. *70:* 300, 1960.

278. *Popper, H., Paronetto, F. & Schaffner, F.:* Immune processes in the pathogenesis of liver disease. Ann. N. Y. Acad. Sci. *124:* 781, 1965.

279. *Popper, H., Rubin, E. & Schaffner, F.:* The problem of primary biliary cirrhosis. Am. J. Med. *33:* 807, 1962.

280. *Popper, H. & Schaffner, F.:* Die Mesenchymreaktion auf Parenchymschädigungen; zum Problem der chronischen Hepatitis. Med. Welt. 1082, 1965.

281. *Popper, H. & Schaffner, F.:* Hepatic cirrhosis, a problem in communication. Isr. J. Med. Sci. *4:* 1, 1968.

282. *Popper, H. & Schaffner, F.:* Pathophysiology of cholestasis. Human Path. *1:* 1, 1970.

283. *Popper, H. & Schaffner, F.:* Nonsuppurative destructive chronic cholangitis and chronic hepatitis. In: Popper, H. & Schaffner, F. (ed.): Progress in Liver Diseases. Vol. 3. New York: Grune & Stratton, p. 336, 1970.

284. *Popper, H. & Thomas, L. B.:* Alterations of liver and spleen among workers exposed to vinyl chlorid. Ann. N. Y. Acad. Sci. (in press).

285. *Popper, H. & Undenfriend, S.:* Hepatic fibrosis: Correlation of biochemical and morphological investigations. Am. J. Med. *49:* 707, 1970.

286. *Porta, E. A., Bergmann, B. J. & Stein, A. A.:* Acute alcoholic hepatitis. Am. J. Path. *46:* 657, 1965.

287. *Porta, E. A. & Hartroft, W. S.:* Lipid pigments in relation of aging and dietary factors (lipofuscins). In: Wolman, M. (ed.): Pigments in Pathology. New York & London: Academic Press. 1969.

288. *Portmann, B., Galbraith, R. M., Eddleston, A. L. F., Zuckerman, A. J. & Williams, R.:* Detection of HB$_S$Ag in fixed liver tissue – use of a modified immunofluorescent technique and comparison with histochemical methods. GUT *17:* 1, 1976.

289. *Poulsen, H.:* Histological features of acute viral hepatitis. Ann. Clin. Res. *8:* 139, 1976.

290. *Poulsen, H. & Christoffersen P.:* Abnormal bile duct epithelium in liver biopsies with histological signs of viral hepatitis. Acta path. microbiol. scand. *76:* 383, 1969.

291. *Poulsen, H. & Christoffersen, P.:* Histological changes in liver biopsies from patients with surgical bile duct disorders. Acta path. microbiol. scand. Section A. *78:* 571, 1970.

292. *Poulsen, H. & Christoffersen, P.:* Abnormal bile duct epithelium in chronic aggressive hepatitis and cirrhosis. Human path. *3:* 217, 1972.

293. *Poulsen, H. & Christoffersen, P.:* Histologische Merkmale der cholestatischen Leber. Euromed. *18:* 198, 1978.

294. *Poulsen, H., Christoffersen, P., Dietrichson, O. & Faber, V.:* The occurrence and significance of abnormal bile duct epithelium in cirrhosis. Acta path. microbiol. scand. Section A. *80:* 659, 1972.

295. *Poulsen, H., Winkler, K. & Christoffersen, P.:* The significance of centrilobular sinusoidal changes in liver biopsies. Scand. J. Gastroent. Suppl. *7:* 103, 1970.

296. *Pyrtek, L. J. & Bartus, S. A.:* Hepatic pyemia. N. Engl. J. Med. *272:* 551, 1965.

297. *Ramalingaswami, V. & Nayak, N. C.:* Liver Disease in India. In: Popper, H. & Schaffner, F. (ed.): Progress in liver Diseases, Vol. 3, New York. Grune & Stratton, p. 222, 1970.

298. *Ranek, L.:* Quantitation of size and composition of liver cell nuclei in acute viral hepatitis. In: Weibel, E. R. (ed.): The Liver. Quantitative Aspects of Structure and Function. Basel: Karger, p. 62, 1973.

299. *Rappaport, A. M.:* Anatomic considerations. In: Schiff, L. (ed.): Diseases of the liver, 4th ed. Philadelphia: Lippincott, p. 1, 1975.

300. *Rappaport, A. M.:* The microcirculatory acinar concept of normal and pathological hepatic structure. Beitr. Pathol. *157:* 215, 1976.

301. *Rappaport, A. M., Boroway, Z. J., Lougheed, W. M. & Lotto, W. N.:* Subdivision of hexagonal liver lobules into a structural and functional unit. Anat. Rec. *119:* 11, 1954.

302. *Ray, M. B. & Desmet, V. J.:* Immunofluorescent detection of hepatitis B antigen in paraffin embedded liver tissue. J. Immun. Meth. *6:* 283, 1975.

303. *Reintoft, I.:* Alpha-l-antitrypsin deficiency. Experience from an autopsy material. Acta path. microbiol. scand. Section A. *85:* 649, 1977.

304. *Reynolds, T. B. & Peters, R. L.:* Budd-Chiari Syndrome. In: Schiff, L. (ed.): Diseases of the Liver, 4th ed. Philadelphia: Lippincott, p. 1402, 1975.

305. *Ritland, S., Steinnes, E. & Skrede, S.:* Hepatic copper content, urinary copper excretion, and serum ceruloplasmin in liver disease. Scand. J. Gastroent. *12:* 81, 1977.

306. *Rozental, P., Biava, C., Spencer, H. & Zimmerman, H. J.:* Liver morphology and function tests in obesity and during total starvation. Am. J. Dig. Dis. *12:* 198, 1967.

307. *Rubin, E.:* Interpretation of liver biopsy. Gastroenterology *45:* 400, 1963.

308. *Rubin, E. & Lieber, C. S.:* The effects of ethanol on the liver. In: Richter, G. W. & Epstein, M. A. (ed.): International Review of Experimental Pathology. New York – London: Academic Press, p. 177, 1972.

309. *Rubin, E. & Popper, H.:* The evolution of human cirrhosis deduced from observations in experimental animals. Medicine *46:* 163, 1967.

310. *Rubin, E., Schaffner, F. & Popper, H.:* Primary biliary cirrhosis. Chronic non-suppurative destructive cholangitis. Am. J. Path. *46:* 387, 1965.

311. *Ruebner, B. H. & Slusser, R. J.:* Hepatocytes and sinusoidal lining cells in viral hepatitis; an electron microscopic study. Arch. Path. *86:* 1, 1968.

312. *Rüttner, J. R. & Vogel, A.:* Elektronenmikroskopische Untersuchungen an der Lebersinusoidwand. Verh. Deutsch. Ges. Path. *41:* 314, 1957.

313. *Salaspuro, M. P. & Sipponen, P.:* Demonstration of an intracellular copperbinding protein by orcein staining in longstanding cholestatic liver diseases. GUT *17:* 787, 1976.

314. *Salaspuro, M. P., Sipponen, P. & Makkonen, H.:* The occurrence of orceinpositive hepatocellular material in various liver diseases. Scand. J. Gastroent. *11:* 677, 1976.

315. *Sama, S. K., Bhargava, S., Gopi Nath, N., Talwar, J. R., Nayak, N. C., Tandon, B. N. & Wig, K. L.:* Non-cirrhotic portal fibrosis. Am. J. Med. *51:* 160, 1971.

316. *Sandritter, W. & Riede, U. N.:* Morphology of liver cell necrosis. In: Keppler, E. (ed.): Pathogenesis and Mechanisms of Liver Cell Necrosis. Lancaster: MTP Press Ltd., p. 1, 1975.

317. *Schaffner, F.:* Intralobular changes in hepatocytes and the electron microscopic mesenchymal response in viral hepatitis. Medicine *45:* 547, 1966.

318. *Schaffner, F., Bacchin, P., Hutterer, F., Scharnbeck, H., Sarkozi, L., Denk, H. & Popper, H.:* Mechanism of cholestasis. IV. Structural and biochemical changes in the liver and serum in rats after bile duct ligation. Gastroenterology *60:* 888, 1971.

319. *Schaffner, F. & Popper, H.:* Non-specific reactive hepatitis in aged and infirm people. Am. J. Dig. Dis. *4:* 389, 1959.

320. *Schaffner, F. & Popper, H.:* Morphologic studies in neonatal cholestasis with emphasis on giant cells. Ann. N. Y. Acad. Sci. *111:* 358, 1963.

321. *Schaffner, F. & Popper, H.:* Electron microscopy of the liver. In: Schiff, L. (ed.): Diseases of the Liver. 4th ed. Philadelphia: Lippincott, p. 51, 1975.

322. *Schaffner, F., Popper, H. & Chesrow, E.:* Cholestasis produced by the administration of norethandrolone. Am. J. Med. *26:* 249, 1959.

323. *Schaffner, F., Sternlieb, I., Barka, T. & Popper, H.:* Hepatocellular changes in Wilson's disease. Am. J. Path. *41:* 315, 1962.

324. *Scheinberg, I. H. & Sternlieb, I.:* Copper metabolism. Pharmacol. Rev. *12:* 355, 1960.

325. *Scheuer, P. J.:* Primary biliary cirrhosis. Proc. R. Soc. Med. *60:* 1257, 1967.

326. *Scheuer, P. J.:* Liver biopsy in the diagnosis of cirrhosis. GUT, *11:* 275, 1970.

327. *Scheuer, P. J.:* Liver biopsy interpretation. 2nd ed. London: Balliére, pp. 21[a], 23[b], 25[c], 26[d], 29[e], 31[f], 41[g], 101[h], 103[i], 123[j], 128[k], 1973.

328. *Scheuer, P. J., Williams, R. & Muir, A. R.:* Hepatic pathology in relatives of patients with haemochromatosis. J. Path. Bact. *84:* 53, 1962.

329. *Schiller, W.:* Local myelopoiesis in myeloid leukemia. Am. J. Path. *19:* 809, 1943.

330. *Schmid, M.:* Die chronische Hepatitis. Berlin: Springer-Verlag. 1966.

331. *Schmid, M. & Cueni, B.:* Portal lesions in viral hepatitis with submassive hepatic necrosis. Human Path. *3:* 209, 1972.

332. *Schubert, W. K.:* Liver disease in infancy and childhood. In: Schiff, L., (ed.): Diseases of the Liver. 4th ed. Philadelphia: Lippincott, p. 1173, 1975.

333. *Scott, J., Summerfield, J. A., Elias, E., Dick, R. & Sherlock, S.:* Chronic pancreatitis: A cause of cholestasis. GUT: *18:* 196, 1977.

334. *Selmair, H. & John, H. D.:* Klinik und Pathologie der Thorotrast. Med. Welt *26:* 1203, 1970.

335. *Sestoft, L., Poulsen, H. & Winkler, K.:* Collagen disease debuting as acute hepatitis. Scand. J. Gastroent. *6:* 495, 1971.

336. *Sharp, H. L. & Freier, E.:* Alpha-l-antitrypsin and familial cirrhosis. Gastroenterology *60:* 179, 1971.

337. *Sharp, H. L., Mathis, R., Krivit, W. & Freier, E.:* The liver in non-cirrhotic alpha-l-antitrypsin. J. Lab. Clin. Med. *78:* 1012, 1971.

338. *Sherlock, S.:* The liver in heart failure; relation of anatomical, functional and circulatory changes. Brit. Heart J. *13:* 273, 1951.

339. *Sherlock, S.:* Portal hypertension. In: Popper, H. & Schaffner, F. (ed.): Progress in Liver Diseases. Vol. 1. New York: Grune & Stratton, p. 145, 1961.

340. *Sherlock, S.:* Chronic cholangitides: aetiology, diagnosis, and treatment. Brit. med. J. *3:* 515, 1968.

341. *Sherlock, S.:* Immunology of liver disease. Am. J. Med. *49:* 693, 1970.

342. *Sherlock, S.:* The liver in circulatory failure. In: Schiff, L. (ed.): Diseases of the Liver. 4th ed. Philadelphia: Lippincott, p. 1033, 1975.

343. *Sherlock, S.:* Diseases of the Liver and Biliary System. 5th ed. Oxford: Blackwell Scientific Publ., p. 445, 1975.

344. *Sherlock, S., Fox, R. A., Niazi, S. P. & Scheuer, P. J.:* Chronic liver disease and primary liver-cell cancer with hepatitisassociated (Australia) antigen in serum. Lancet *i:* 1243, 1970.

345. *Shikata, T.:* Australia antigen in hepatoma and cirrhosis tissue. Tumor Res. *8:* 127, 1973.

346. *Shikata, T., Uzawa, T., Yoshiwara, N., Akatsuka, T. & Yamazaki, S.:* Staining methods of Australia antigen in paraffin section – detection of cytoplasmic inclusion bodies. Jap. J. Exp. Med. *44:* 25, 1974.

347. *Sipponen, P., Salaspuro, M. P. & Makkonen, H. M.:* Orcein-positive hepatocellular material in histological diagnosis of primary biliary cirrhosis. Ann. Clin. Res. *7:* 273, 1975.

348. *Smetana, H. F.:* Pathologic anatomy of early stages of viral hepatitis. In: Hartman, F., Lo Grippo, G. A., Mateer, J. G. & Barron, J. (ed.): Hepatitis Frontiers. Boston: Brown & Co. p. 77, 1957.

349. *Smetana, H. F., Hadley, G. G. & Sirsat, S. M.:* Infantile cirrhosis. Pediatrics *28:* 107, 1961.

350. *Smetana, H. F. & Olen, E.:* Hereditary galactose disease. Am. J. Clin. Path. *38:* 3, 1962.

351. *Sobel, H. J., Schwarz, R. & Marquet, E.:* Non-viral nuclear inclusions. 2. Glykogen and lipid. Lab. Invest. *20:* 604, 1969.

352. *Soloway, R. D., Baggenstoss, A. H., Schoenfield, L. J. & Summerskill, W. H. J.:* Observer error and sampling variability tested in evaluation of hepatitis and cirrhosis by liver biopsy. Am. J. Dig. Dis. *16:* 1082, 1971.

353. *Soloway, R. D., Summerskill, W. H. J., Baggenstoss, A. H., Geall, M. G., Gitnick, G. L., Elveback, L. R. & Schoenfield, L. J.:* Clinical, biochemical and histological remission of severe chronic active liver disease: a controlled study of treatments and early prognosis. Gastroenterology, *63:* 820, 1972.

354. *Sparrow, W. T. & Ashworth, C. T.:* Electron microscopy of nuclear glycogenesis. Arch. Path. *80:* 84, 1965.

355. *Starup, K. & Mosbeck, J.:* Budd-Chiari syndrome after taking oral contraceptives. Brit. Med. J. *4:* 660, 1967.

356. *Staubli, W., Hess, R. & Weibel, E. R.:* Correlated morphometric and biochemical studies on the liver cell. II. Effects of phenobarbital on rat hepatocytes. J. Cell. Biol. *42:* 92, 1969.

357. *Stauffer, M. H., Gross, J. B., Foulk, W. T. & Dahlin, D. C.:* Amyloidosis: Diagnosis with needle biopsy of the liver in eighteen patients. Gastroenterology *41:* 92, 1961.

358. *Steiner, J. W. & Carruthers, J. S.:* Studies on the fine structure of the terminal branches of the biliary tree. I: The morphology of normal bile canaliculi, preductules and bile ductules. Am. J. Path. *38:* 639, 1961.

359. *Steiner, J. W. & Carruthers, J. S.:* Experimental extrahepatic biliary obstruction. Some aspects of the fine structural changes of bile ductules and preductules (ducts of Hering). Am. J. Path. *40:* 253, 1962.

360. *Steiner, P. E.:* Nodular regenerative hyperplasia of the liver. Am. J. Path. *35:* 943, 1959.

361. *Sternlieb, I.:* Mitochrondrial and fatty changes in hepatocytes of patients with Wilson's disease. Gastroenterology *55:* 354, 1968.

362. *Sternlieb, I. & Scheinberg, I. H.:* Chronic hepatitis as a first manifestation of Wilson's disease. Ann. intern. Med. *76:* 59, 1972.

363. *Stockinger, L.:* Disséscher Raum und Bindegewebszelle in der menschlichen Leber. Ergh. Anat. Anz. *120:* 545, 1966.

364. *Stone, W. D., Islam, N. R. K. & Paton, A.:* The natural history of cirrhosis. Quart. J. Med. *37:* 119, 1968.

365. *Sunzel, H. L. & Zettergren, L.:* Histological liver lesions developing during abdominal operations. Gastroenterologia *105:* 45, 1966.

366. *Symmers, W. St. C.:* Primary amyloidosis. A review. J. Clin. Path. *9:* 187, 1956.

367. *Tajiri, S.:* The terminal distribution of the hepatic artery. Acta. Med. Okayama. *14:* 215, 1960.

368. *Thaler, H.:* Leberbiopsie. Berlin: Springer-Verlag, p. 140, 1969.

369. *Thomas, L. B. & Popper, H.:* Pathology of angiosarcoma of the liver in vinyl chloride-polyvinyl chloride workers. Ann. NY. Acad. Sci. *246:* 268, 1975.

370. *Thomas, D. B., Russel, P. M. & Yoffey, J. M.:* Pattern of hematopoiesis in fetal liver. Nature *187:* 876, 1960.

371. *Thommesen, N.:* Biliary hamartomas (von Meyenburg Complexes) in liver needle biopsies. Acta path. microbiol. scand. Section A. *86:* 93, 1978.

372. *Thomsen, P., Poulsen, H. & Petersen, P.:* Different types of ground glass hepatocytes in human liver biopsies; morphology, occurrence and diagnostic significance. Scand. J. Gastr. *11:* 113, 1976

373. *Thorpe, M. E. C., Scheuer, P. J. & Sherlock, S.:* Primary sclerosing cholangitis, the biliary tree, and ulcerative colitis. GUT *8:* 435, 1967.

374. *Tinney, W. S., Hall, B. E. & Griffin, H. Z.:* The liver and spleen in polycythemia vera. Proc. Staff Meet. Mayo Clin. *18:* 46, 1943.

375. *Tisdale, W. A.:* Clinical and pathologic features of subacute hepatitis. Medicine *45:* 557, 1966.

376. *Torres, A.:* Primary lymphocytic follicular lymphoma of liver. Cancer *23:* 1185, 1969.

377. *Torres, A. & Bollozos, G. D.:* Primary reticulum cell sarcoma of the liver. Cancer *27:* 1489, 1971.

378. *Trepo, C. & Thivolet, J.:* Antigene Australia, hepatic virale et periarterite nodeuse. Nouvelle Presse Médicale *78:* 1575, 1970.

379. *Triger, D. R.:* The liver as an immunological organ. Gastroenterology *71:* 162, 1976.

380. *U. S. Government Printing Office:* Diseases of the Liver and Biliary tract. Standardization of Nomenclature, Diagnostic Criteria and Diagnostic Methodology. Washington, Fogarty International Center Proceedings, N° 22. Washington: DHEW Publication (NIH) 76–725, 1976.

381. *Valman, H. B., France, N. E. & Wallis, P. G.:* Prolonged neonatal jaundice in cystic fibrosis. Arch. Dis. Childh. *46:* 805, 1971.

382. *Vido, L., Selmair, E., Wildhirt, E. & Ortmans, H.:* Zur Prognose der chronischen Hepatitis. I. Formen und Entwicklungsstadien. Dtsch. med. Wschr. *94:* 2215, 1969.

383. *Vischer, T. L., Bernheim, C. & Engelbrect, E.:* Two cases of hepatitis due to Toxoplasma gondii. Lancet *ii:* 919, 1967.

384. *Visfeldt, J. & Poulsen, H.:* On the histopathology of liver and liver tumours in thorium-dioxide patients. Acta path. microbiol. scand. Section A. *80:* 97, 1972.

385. *Volk, B. J. & Wallace, B. J.:* The liver in lipidosis. An electron microscopic and histochemical study. Am. J. Path. *49:* 203, 1966.

386. *von Kupffer, C.:* Über die sogenannten Sternzellen der Säugertierleber. Arch. Mikr. Anat. Entwicklungsgesch. *54:* 254, 1899.

387. *Wadsworth, R. C. & Keil, P. G.:* Biopsy of the liver in infectious mononucleosis. Am. J. Path. *28:* 1003, 1952.

388. *Waldstein, S. S. & Szanto, P. B.:* Accuracy of sampling by needle biopsy in diffuse liver disease. Arch. Path. *50:* 326, 1950.

389. *Walker, R. J., Miller, J. P. G., Dymock, I. W., Shilken, K. B. & Williams, R.:* Relationship of hepatic iron concentration to histochemical grading and to total chelatable body iron in conditions associated with iron overload. GUT *12:* 1011, 1971.

390. *Wallach, H. F. & Popper, H.:* Central necrosis of the liver. Arch. Path. *49:* 33, 1950.

391. *Warren, K. S.:* Hepatosplenic schistosomiasis mansoni: An immunologic disease. Bull. N. Y. Acad. Med. *51:* 545, 1975.

392. *Wassermann, F.:* The structure of the wall of the hepatic sinusoids in the electron microscope. Z. Zellforsch. *49:* 13, 1958.

393. *Williams, R., Williams, H. S., Scheuer, P. J., Pitcher, C. S., Loiseau, E. & Sherlock, S.:* Iron absorption and siderosis in chronic liver disease. Quart. J. Med. *36:* 151, 1967.

394. *Wilson, J. W., Groat, C. S. & Leduc, E. H.:* Histogenesis of the liver. Ann. N. Y. Acad. Sci. *111:* 8, 1963.

395. *Winkler. K. & Poulsen, H.:* Liver disease with periportal sinusoidal dilatation. Scand. J. Gastroent. *10:* 699, 1975.

396. *Woehler, F.:* Ferritin and haemosiderin. Germ. Med. Mth. *9:* 377, 1964.

397. *Wohlgemuth, B. & Reichmann, J.:* Histomorphologische Leberbefunde beim Gastroduodenalulcus. Acta Hepatosplen. (Stuttgart) *12:* 65, 1965.

398. *Wood, R. L.:* The fine structure of the junction between bile canaliculi and bile ducts in mammalian liver. Anat. Rec. *139:* 287, 1961.

399. *Yanoff, M. & Rawson, A. J.:* Peliosis hepatis. Arch. Path. *77:* 159, 1964.

400. *Zeek, P. M.:* Periarteritis nodosa. A critical review. Am. J. Clin. Path. *22:* 777, 1952.

401. *Zelman, S.:* Liver cell necrosis in chlorpromazine jaundice. Am. J. Med. *27:* 708, 1959.

402. *Zimmerman, H. J. & Thomas, L. J.:* The liver in pneumococcal pneumonia: Observation in 94 cases on liver function and jaundice in pneumonia. J. Lab. Clin. Med. *35:* 556, 1950.

403. *Zollinger, H. U.:* Trübe Schwellung und Mitochondrien. Schweiz. Z. Pathol. *11:* 617, 1948.

General Reading

Becker, F. F. (ed.): The Liver. Normal and Abnormal Functions. New York: Marcel Dekker. 1975.

Bianchi, L.: Punktat-Morphologie und Differentialdiagnose der Hepatitis. Stuttgart: Hans Huber Verlag, 1967.

Bolck, F. & Machnik, G.: Leber und Gallenwege. In: Doerr, W., Seifert, G. & Uehlinger, E. (ed.): Spezielle pathologische Anatomie. Band 10. Berlin-Heidelberg-New York: Springer Verlag, 1978.

Edmondson, H. A.: Tumors of the liver and intrahepatic bile ducts. Atlas of Tumor Pathology, Section VII, Fascicle 25. Washington: A. F. I. P. 1958.

Elias, H. & Sherrick, J. C.: Morphology of the Liver. New York: Academic Press. 1969.

Gall, E. A. & Mostofi, F. K. (ed.): The Liver. International Academy of Pathology. Monograph 13. Baltimore: Williams & Wilkins. 1973.

Gerok, W. & Sickinger, K. (ed.): Drugs and the Liver. Stuttgart: Schattauer Verlag, 1975.

Keppler, D. (ed.): Pathogenesis and Mechanism of Liver Cell Necrosis. Lancaster: MTP Press. 1975.

Okuda, K. & Peters, R. L. (ed.): Hepatocellular Carcinoma. New York: John Wiley & Sons, 1976.

Popper, H. (ed.): Cirrhosis. Clinics in Gastroenterology. Vol. 4. Philadelphia: Saunders. 1975.

Popper, H. & Schaffner, F.: Liver: Structure and Function. New York: McGraw-Hill Book Co., 1957.

Popper, H. & Schaffner, F. (ed.): Progress in Liver Diseases. Vol. 1–5. New York: Grune & Stratton. 1969–1976.

Schaffner, F., Sherlock, S. & Leevy, C. M. (ed.): The Liver and Its Diseases. Stuttgart: Thieme. 1974.

Scheuer, P. J.: Liver Biopsy Interpretation, 2nd ed. London: Bailliére. 1973.

Schmid, M.: Die chronische Hepatitis. Berlin: Springer-Verlag 1966.

Sherlock, S.: Diseases of the Liver and Biliary System. 5th ed. Oxford: Blackwell Scientific Publ. 1975.

Schiff, L. (ed.): Diseases of the Liver, 4th ed. Philadelphia: Lippincott. 1975.

Shorter, R. G.: Liver Biopsy. An Atlas of Histologic Apperances. Oxford: Pergamon Press. 1961.

Thaler, H.: Leberbiopsie. Berlin: Springer-Verlag. 1969.

Tygstrup, N. (ed.): Viral Hepatitis. Clinics in Gastroenterology, Vol. 3. Philadelphia: Saunders. 1974.

U. S. Goverment Printing Office: Diseases of the Liver and Biliary Tract. Standardization of Nomenclature, Diagnostic Criteria and Diagnostic Methodology. Washington, Fogarty International Center Proceedings, N° 22. Washington: DHEW Publication (NIH) 76–725, 1976.

Wallnöfer, H., Schmidt, E. & Schmidt, F. W.: Diagnosis of Liver Diseases. Stuttgart: Thieme Verlag, 1977.

Wepler, W. & Wildhirt, E.: Klinische Histopathologie der Leber. Stuttgart: Thieme Verlag, 1968.

Technical Appendix

In this appendix* we have described the processing schedule and staining methods used in our laboratory for light microscopy of liver biopsies. The methods chosen are in our experience the best for routine diagnostic work and form the basis of the histopathological description given in chapters 2 and 3. We have attempted to give sufficient details to make it possible to reproduce our results.

With regard to staining methods we have in principle followed the text of *Histopathologic Technic and Practical Histochemistry* by R. D. Lillie and H. M. Fullmer (1976). In the few exceptions to this we have given the full reference to the original paper under the method in question. As the staining methods have all been modified to some degree, however, they are given in full and should, if fixation, dehydration, paraffin embedding and sectioning are in accordance with the specifications given below, lead to the results we have found desirable. All reagents apart from stains should be of analytical reagent grade, unless otherwise specified. For stains the C. I. (Color Index) numbers have been given.

As several of the stains may vary in composition from batch to batch and from different manufacturers, it is necessary, when using the majority of the staining methods, to include control sections for purposes of reference. When not otherwise specified solutions are prepared with distilled water. For the individual staining methods the most characteristic features are given as "results" so as to enable a microscopic evaluation of the staining reaction in the laboratory.

* Written in collaboration with Hans Lyon M.D.

Fixation and Embedding

Immediately after the liver biopsy has been performed, it is placed in neutral buffered formaldehyde solution at room temperature for 1–3 hours.

NEUTRAL BUFFERED FORMALDEHYDE SOLUTION, 36 g/l

Formaldehyde (HCHO, M_r = 30.0) 360 g/l	100 ml
Distilled water	900 ml
Sodium dihydrogenphosphate (NaH_2PO_4, H_2O, M_r = 138.0)	4 g
Anhydrous disodium hydrogenphosphate (Na_2HPO_4, M_r = 142.0)	6.5 g

DEHYDRATION AND PARAFFIN INFILTRATION
After fixation the biopsies are dehydrated and infiltrated with paraffin in a tissue processing machine according to the following schedule:

Dehydration and paraffin infiltration procedure:

Bath	Solution	Time
1	Neutral buffered formaldehyde solution, pH 7, 36 g/l	15 min
2	70% w/v ethanol	15 min
3	93% w/v ethanol	15 min
4	99% w/v ethanol	15 min
5	Xylene (mixture of the three isomers), M_r = 106.2	15 min
6	Xylene-paraffin 1+1 (60°C)	15 min
7	Paraffin (60°C)	15 min
8	Paraffin (60°C)	15 min

The biopsies are then embedded in paraffin. We currently use Paraplast®. A total of 54 sections are cut on a rotary microtome set at 5 μm. After the sections have been spread on a warm-water bath, they are consecutively floated on clean slides, three sections on each slide.

Staining of Slides

Staining of the slides is performed according to the following schedule (see Fig. 6), and the detailed procedures follow in the same order as here:

Slide no.	Section no.	Staining procedure	Chief diagnostic advantage
1	1- 2- 3	Hematoxylin and Eosin	General oversight
2	4- 5- 6	van Gieson's stain	Bile thrombi and collagen
3	7- 8- 9	Masson's trichrome stain	Collagen and reticulin
4	10–11–12	Hematoxylin and Eosin	
5	13–14–15	Silver impregnation	Reticulin
6	16–17–18	Rhodanine stain or rubeanic acid stain	Copper deposits
7	19–20–21	Hematoxylin and Eosin	
8	22–23–24	Periodic acid Schiff reaction (PAS)	PAS-positive components
9	25–26–27	PAS reaction following saliva digestion	PAS-positive components except glycogen
10	28–29–30	van Gieson's stain	
11	31–32–33	Methyl green Pyronin	RNA
12	34–35–36	Hematoxylin and Eosin	
13	37–38–39	van Gieson's stain	
14	40–41–42	Ferrocyanide reaction	Hemosiderin deposits
15	43–44–45	Hematoxylin and Eosin	
16	46–47–48	Silver impregnation	
17	49–50–51	van Gieson's stain	
18	52–53–54	Orcein staining	HB_SAg and copper deposits

Hematoxylin and Eosin

Staining solutions:

Mayer's alum hematoxylin

Hematoxylin ($C_{16}H_{14}O_6 \cdot 3H_2O$ C. I. 75290, M_r = 356.3)	1 g
Distilled water	1000 ml
Sodium iodate ($NaIO_3$, M_r = 197.9)	0.2 g
Ammonium aluminum (ammonium alum, $Al_2(SO_4)_3$, $(NH_4)_2SO_4$, 24 H_2O, M_r = 906.71)	50 g

After water has been added to the hematoxylin, the solution is gently heated until all the hematoxylin is dissolved. The sodium iodate is added and when this is completely dissolved, indicated by the solution becoming reddish, the ammonium alum is added. The staining solution is immediately ready for use.

Eosin

Eosin (eosin Y) (C.I. 45380)	1 g
Distilled water	100 ml

Staining procedure:

Bring section to water.

1. Stain sections in Mayer's alum hematoxylin	10 min
2. Wash in running tap water	
3. Stain in aqueous eosin 1 g/l	5 min
4. Dehydrate with two changes each of 95% w/v and 99% w/v alcohol	
5. Pass through two changes of xylene	
6. Mount in synthetic resin	

Results:

Nuclei blue; cytoplasm and collagen varying shades of pink.

Van Gieson's stain

Staining solutions:	*Weigert-Lillie stabilized iron chloride hematoxylin*	
	A. Ferric chloride ($FeCl_3$. $6H_2O$, M_r = 270.3) 25 g/l	100 ml
	Ferrous sulfate ($FeSO_4$. $7H_2O$, M_r = 278.0) 45 g/l	100 ml
	Concentrated hydrochloric acid (HCl, M_r = 36.5) 13.1 mol/l	98 ml
	B. Hematoxylin ($C_{16}H_{14}O_6$. $3H_2O$, C.I. 75290, M_r = 356.3)	1 g
	Ethanol, anhydrous	100 ml

Final staining solution: A and B are mixed (3 volumens A to 1 volume B). We prepare fresh mixtures every second or third day.

Picrofuschsin stain

Aqueous picric acid solution (2,4,6-trinitro-phenol, $C_6H_3N_3O_7$, C.I. 10305, M_r = 229.1) 12 g/l	940 ml
Acid fuchsin (C.I. 42685), 20 g/l	50 ml
Glacial acetic acid (CH_3COOH, M_r = 60.0) 17.4 mol/l	10 ml

Staining procedure: Bring sections to water.

1. Stain with Weigert-Lillie stabilized iron chloride hematoxylin for 8 min
2. Wash 5 min in running water
3. Stain 5 min in picrofuschsin mixture
4. Very short rinse in running tap water
5. Dehydrate in two changes each of 95% w/v and 100% w/v alcohol
6. Clear in two changes of pure xylene. Mount in resin.

Results: Collagen fibers red (compare text p. 150); cytoplasm of hepatocytes grey; erythrocytes and smooth muscle cells yellow; nuclei brown-black.

Silver Impregnation for Reticulin Fibers

Staining solutions:

Acidified permanganate solution

Potassium permanganate ($KMnO_4$, $M_r = 158.0$) 5 g/l	190 ml
Sulfuric acid (H_2SO_4, $M_r = 98.1$) 3.1×10^{-1} mol/l	10 ml

The sulfuric acid is added immediately before use.

Oxalic acid $((COOH)_2, 2H_2O, M_r = 90.0)$	1 g
Distilled water	100 ml

Iron alum

Ammonium iron sulfate (Iron alum, $Fe_2(SO_4)_3$, $(NH_4)_2$, $24H_2O$, $M_r = 964.4$)	2.5 g
Distilled water	100 ml

Silver solution

Silver nitrate ($AgNO_3$, $M_r = 169.9$)	100 g/l
Ammonia water (NH_3, $M_r = 17.0$)	280 g/l
Sodium hydroxide ($NaOH$, $M_r = 40.0$)	30 g/l

To 20 ml aqueous silver nitrate 100 g/l add ammonia water 280 g/l drop by drop under constant shaking until the solution is clear.

20 ml sodium hydroxide 30 g/l is added. Ammonia is again added until the precipitate is dissolved. Make up to 200 ml with distilled water.

Aqueous formaldehyde

Formaldehyde ($HCHO$, $M_r = 30.0$) 360 g/l	100 ml
Distilled water	900 ml

Gold chloride

Hydrogen tetrachloroaurate (acid gold trichloride, $HAuCl_4$, $M_r = 339.8$)	0.2 g
Distilled water	100 ml

Sodium thiosulfate

Sodium thiosulfate ($Na_2S_2O_3 . 5H_2O$, $M_r = 248.3$)	2.5 g
Distilled water	100 ml

(continued)

Silver Impregnation for Reticulin Fibers
(continued)

Staining procedure:	Bring sections to water.	
	1. Oxidize in acidified permanganate solution	3 min
	2. Running tap water	5 min
	3. Bleach in oxalic acid 1×10^{-1} mol/l	1 min
	4. Running tap water	5 min
	5. Mordant in aqueous iron alum 25 g/l	15 min
	6. Wash in two changes of distilled water	
	7. Treat with silver solution	30 s
	8. Wash in four or five changes of distilled water	
	9. Reduce in aqueous formaldehyde 36 g/l	30 s
	10. Running tap water	5 min
	11. Tone in gold chloride 2 g/l	1 min
	12. Wash in two changes of distilled water	
	13. Fix in sodium thiosulfate 25 g/l	5 min
	14. Running tap water	5 min
	15. Dehydration through graded alcohols, xylene, synthetic resin.	

Note that the process is irreversible from step 11. The sections should therefore be examined immediately prior to this step, and in case of unsatisfactory impregnation, the process may be repeated from step 5.

Results: Reticulin fibers black; collagen fibers pale grey; elastic fibers jet black; background almost colorless.

Reference: *Gordon, H. & Sweets, Jr., H. H.:* A simple method for the silver impregnation of reticulum. Am. J. Pathol. *12,* 545–551, 1936.

Rhodanine Stain for Copper

Staining solutions:

Saturated rhodanine solution (stock 2 g/l)

5-(4-dimethylaminobenzyliden)-rhodanine ($C_{12}H_{12}N_2OS_2$, M_r = 264.4)	0.2 g
Ethanol, anhydrous	100 ml

Rhodanine working solution (0.12 g/l)

Saturated rhodanine solution	6 ml
Distilled water	94 ml

The saturated rhodanine solution should be shaken vigorously before measuring and mixing solutions.

Diluted Mayer's alum hematoxylin

Mayer's alum hematoxylin (see p. 222)	50 ml
Distilled water	50 ml

Sodium tetraborate solution (5 g/l)

Sodium tetraborate decahydrate (borax) ($Na_2B_4O_7 \cdot 10H_2O$, M_r = 381.4)	0.5 g
Distilled water	100 ml

Staining procedure:

Bring sections to water.

1. Incubate in rhodanine working solution at 37°C	18 h
2. Wash well in several changes of distilled water	
3. Stain in diluted Mayer's alum hematoxylin	10 min
4. Rinse with distilled water	
5. Rinse in sodium tetraborate solution for five 1 s dips	
6. Rinse well with distilled water	
7. Dehydrate in two changes each of 95% w/v and 100% w/v alcohol. Clear in two changes of xylene. Mount in resin.	

Results:

Copper deposits bright red (note that the color fades over a period of days). Background light blue.

References:

Lindquist, R. R.: Studies on the pathogenesis of hepatolenticular degeneration. II. Cytochemical methods for the localization of copper. Arch. Path. *87*, 370–379, 1969.

Okamoto, K. & Utamura, M.: Biologische Untersuchungen des Kupffers. Über die histochemische Kupffernachweismethode. Acta. Schol. Med. Univ. Imp. Kioto *20*, 573–580, 1938.

Rubeanic Acid Stain for Copper

Staining solutions:

Rubeanic acid solution (stock 1 g/l)

Rubeanic acid (dithiooxamide, $C_2H_4N_2S_2$, $M_r = 120.2$)	0.1 g
Ethanol, anhydrous	100 ml

Store in refrigerator

Rubeanic acid working solutions (0.05 g/l)

Rubeanic acid stock solution	5 ml
Aqueous sodium acetate (CH_3COONa, $M_r = 82.0$) 100 g/l	100 ml

Neutral red (2 g/l)

Neutral red (C.I. 50040)	0.2 g
Distilled water	100 ml

Staining procedure

Bring sections to water.

1. Incubate in rubeanic acid working solution a 37°C in a tightly covered vessel for 18 h (12–24 h)
2. Wash in distilled water
3. Counterstain with Neutral red for 1 min
4. Blot dry and dehydrate with two changes of 100% w/v alcohol. Clear in two changes of xylene.
5. Mount in resin.

Results:

Copper deposits greenish black; nuclei red.

Periodic Acid Schiff Reaction (PAS)

Staining solutions:

Periodic acid (2×10^{-1} mol/l)

Periodic acid	0.5 g
Distilled water	100 ml

Hydrochloric acid alcohol

70% w/v ethanol	99 ml
Concentrated hydrochloric acid (HCl, $M_r = 36.5$) 13.1 mol/l	1 ml

Schiff's sulfurous acid leucofuchsin reagent

Basic fuchsin (C.I. 42500)	3.75 g
Alcohol, anhydrous	50 ml
Distilled water	450 ml
Potassium pyrosulfite (potassium metabisulfite, $K_2S_2O_5$, $M_r = 222.3$)	3.75 g
Hydrochloric acid 1.0 mol/l	75 ml
Sodium hydrosulfite (sodium dithionite, $Na_2S_2O_4 . 2H_2O$, $M_r = 210.2$)	2.5 g

The basic fuchsin is dissolved in absolute alcohol. Some of the water is added, and the solution is heated until the basic fuchsin is completely dissolved. The rest of the water is added followed by potassium pyrosulfite. When this is dissolved the hydrochloric acid is added followed by sodium hydrosulfite. After standing for 15 min, 8–10 g activated charcoal is added and the solution is shaken vigorously for 5 min, and then filtered.

Mayer's alum hematoxylin (see p. 222).

(continued)

Periodic Acid Schiff Reaction (PAS)

(continued)

Staining procedure:
Bring sections to water.

1. Oxidize for exactly 5 min in periodic acid
2. Wash 5 min in running tap water
3. Immerse for 15 min in Schiff's reagent
4. Wash in hydrochloric acid alcohol for ten 1 s dips
5. Running tap water   5 min
6. Mayer's alum hematoxylin   5 min
7. Running tap water   10 min
8. Dehydrate in two changes each of 95% w/v and 100% w/v alcohol. Clear in two changes of xylene.

   Mount in resin.

Results
PAS-positive components are stained magenta. Among these are glycogen, collagen and reticulin fibres.

PAS REACTION FOLLOWING SALIVA DIGESTION

Reagent:
Saliva

Fresh saliva   1 ml
Distilled water   1 ml

The mixture is centrifuged at 300 G for 10 min. The middle phase (water phase) is removed by means of a pipette and flooded on sections.

Procedure
Bring sections to water.

Sections are placed in the saliva preparation for 30 min at 37°C. After rinsing in water the sections are subjected to the routine PAS reaction (see this).

Results:
The results are as for the PAS reaction with the exception that glycogen is completely removed.

Masson's Trichrome Stain

Staining solutions: Weigert-Lillie stabilized iron chloride hematoxylin (see p. 223).

Ponceau 2R-acid fuchsin

Ponceau 2R (C.I. 16150)	0.6 g
Acid fuchsin (C.I. 42685)	0.3 g
Glacial acetic acid (CH_3COOH, M_r = 60.0) 17.4 mol/l	1 ml
Distilled water	100 ml

Phosphomolybdic acid solution

Phosphomolybdic acid ($H_3(P(Mo_3O_{10})_4)$)	1 g
Distilled water	100 ml

Aniline blue acetic acid

Aniline blue (C.I. 42755)	2.5 g
Glacial acetic acid ($CH_3 COOH$, M_r = 60.0) 17.4 mol/l	2.5 g
Distilled water	100 ml

Staining procedure: Bring sections to water.

1. Stain with Weigert-Lillie stabilized iron chloride hematoxylin for 8 min
2. Wash 5 min in running tap water. Transfer to distilled water
3. Stain 10 min in ponceau 2R-acid fuchsin solution
4. Rinse in three changes of distilled water
5. Mordant 5 min in 1% w/v aqueous phosphomolybdic acid solution Drain, and
6. Stain 5 min in aniline blue acetic acid solution
7. Differentiate 2 min in 1% w/v (1.7×10^{-1} mol/l) acetic acid
8. Dehydrate, clear and mount by a alcohol, xylene, resin sequence.

Results: Collagen and reticulin fibers blue; cytoplasm of hepatocytes granular brownish red; erythrocytes and nucleoli red; nuclei blue-black.

Methyl Green Pyronin

Staining solutions:

Acetate buffer pH 4.8

Acetic acid (CH_3COOH, M_r = 60.0) 0.2 mol/l	60 ml
Sodium acetate (CH_3COONa, M_r = 82.0) 0.2 mol/l	90 ml

Methyl green pyronin solution

Aqueous pyronin (C.I. 45005) solution 30 g/l	17.5 ml
Chloroform extracted aqueous methyl green (C.I. 42585) solution 20 g/l	10 ml
Distilled water	200 ml

Methyl green pyronin solution pH 4.8

Methyl green pyronin solution	50 ml
Acetate buffer pH 4.8	150 ml

Staining procedure:

Bring sections to water

1. Stain in methyl green pyronin solution pH 4.8   15 min
2. Wash in distilled water
3. Blot dry. (The sections must be completely dry)
4. Two changes of acetone; clear through acetone plus xylene (50+50) and two changes of xylene; mount in synthetic resin.

Results:

Nuclei (DNA) blue green; nucleoli (RNA) red; cytoplasm (RNA) red.

Ferrocyanide Reaction for Iron

Staining solutions:	*Potassium ferrocyanide solution*

Potassium ferrocyanide ($K_4Fe(CN)_6$, $3H_2O$, $M_r = 422.4$)   2 g

Hydrochloric acid (HCl, $M_r = 36.5$) 3×10^{-1} mol/l   200 ml

The solution is freshly made up before use.

Hydrochloric acid alcohol

(see PAS reaction)

Schiff's reagent

(see PAS reaction)

Staining procedure: Bring sections to water.

1. Potassium ferrocyanide solution   30 min
2. Rinse in distilled water
3. Hydrolyze in 5 M hydrochloric acid   10 min
4. Two changes of distilled water   2 min
5. Schiff's reagent   15 min
6. Hydrochloric acid alcohol   5 brief (10 s) dips
7. Running tap water   10 min
8. Dehydrate through alcohols; clear in xylene; mount in nonreducing resin.

Note: All glassware should be rinsed in 3×10^{-1} mol/l hydrochloric acid prior to the reaction. The use of utensils containing iron should be avoided throughout the reaction.

Results: Reaction sites are blue or green representing hemosiderin; nuclei (DNA) magenta.

Orcein Stain

Staining solutions:

Acidified potassium permanganate solution

Potassium permanganate ($KMnO_4$, $M_r = 158.0$)	1.5 g
Distilled water	100 ml
Concentrated sulfuric acid (H_SSO_4, $M_r = 98.1$) 18.6 mol/l	

The sulfuric acid is added immediately before use.

Orcein solution

Orcein (C.I. (ed. 1) 1242)	1 g
70% w/v ethanol	100 ml
Concentrated hydrochloric acid (HCl, $M_r = 36.5$) 13.1 mol/l	1 ml

Note:

Synthetic orceins from different manufacturers are not identical in their behavior, and it is quite difficult to obtain batches which give a satisfactory result with this method. We have obtained excellent results with batch no. 2479310 from BDH Chemicals Ltd. Poole, England.

Staining procedure:

Sections to water.

1. Oxidize in acidified permanganate solution   5 min
2. Destain in oxalic acid until sections are pale (about 1 min)
3. Stain with orcein   4 h
4. Dehydrate in two changes of 99% w/v alcohol; clear in two changes of xylene; mount in synthetic resin.

Results:

Hepatitis B antigen (HB_SAg) is stained dark brown; elastic fibers dark brown.

Reference:

Shikata, T., Uzawa, T., Yoshiwara, N., Akatsuka, T. & Yamazaki, S.: Staining methods of Australia antigen in paraffin section – detection of cytoplasmic inclusion bodies. Jap. J. Exp. Med. *44,* 25–36, 1974.

Index*

A

Abnormal bile duct epithelium *see Bile ducts*
Abscess 96
Acidophil bodies *80,* 110, 114, 172, 180, 182
  (23, 68, 69, 171)
Acinus *22,* 26, 90, 146, 160, 162 (11)
Acute hepatitis 54, 58, 66, 70, 72, 80, 82, 84,
  86, 90, 102, 104, 106, 120, 132, 134, 160, 162,
  170, *172–174,* 180, 182, 184 (8, 9, 64, 68, 70, 71,
  74, 75, 76, 77, 78, 79, 92, 93, 114, 150, 157, 158,
  159, 160, 161)
Adenoma *see Hepatocellular adenoma*
Adenomatous proliferation *see Rosettes*
Alcoholic hepatitis 32, 44, 50, *92,* 96, 108, 110,
  120, 154, 156, 160, 186, 190, 192 (80, 81)
Allopurinol 42
Alpha-l-antirypsin deficiency 108, 114
  (102, 103)
Amyloidosis 60, 70, 74, *144* (132, 133)
Anemia 120
Anoxia 96
Architecture *see Lobular architecture*
Arsenic 28, 152
Artefacts 11, 70, 104, 118, 130 (5)
Arteriolosclerosis 60 (48)
Ascending cholangitis 32, 48
Atrophy of liver cell plates *130,* 198
  (58, 118, 119)

B

Ballooning of liver cells 70, *104,* 106, 172
  (92, 93)
Banti's syndrome 152
Barbiturates 56, 118
Beryllosis 42
Bile canaliculi 68, 76, 78
Bile ducts
  abnormal configuration 52 (40, 41)
  abnormal epithelium, hepatitis type *54,* 56,
    174, 176, 190, 192 (42, 43)
  abnormal epithelium, PBC type 54, *56,*
    188, 190, 192 (44, 45)
  decreased number 46 (34, 35, 175)
  proliferation, diffuse *48,* 174, 176, 188, 190,
    192 (31, 37)

  proliferation, marginal 32, *50,* 56, 186, 188
    (21, 33, 34, 38, 39, 54, 55, 172)
Bile ductules 30
Bile infarct 98, 106 (86, 87)
Bile lake 98 (46)
Bile pigment *58,* 126, 134 (65, 114, 122)
Bile thrombi *see Cholestasis*
Biliary atresia 46, 50
Biopsy
  adequacy of 16–18
  chemical analysis 12
  electron microscopy 12, 16
  embedding 14
  fixation 14
  frozen sections 12
  initial treatment 12
  naked eye appearance 11 (1–4)
  needle, types of 10, 11
  sectioning 14
  stains for routine 14, 16
  stain procedures *see Technical appendix*
  surgical 11
Bridging fibrosis 156, *162,* 176 (149, 150, 151,
  162, 163)
Bridging necrosis 86, *90,* 174, 176, 192 (78, 79)
Brucellosis 36, 42
Budd-Chiari's syndrome *148,* 198
  (136, 137, 185)
By-pass operation 92

C

Canaliculi *see Bile canaliculi*
Canals of Hering 30
Capsule 150 (138)
Carbon 40, 58, 134
Carbon tetrachloride 86
Carcinoma *see Hepatocellular Carcinoma*
Cardiac cirrhosis 198
Cardiac shock 86, 148, 160, 198 (148, 184)
Caroli's disease 52
Central hyaline sclerosis 92, 110, 156, *160,* 190
  (149)
Central vein *see Hepatic vein radicles*
Centrilobular fibrosis 160 (148, 149)

---

* Principal references are indicated by italicized numerals and numbers in brackets refer to illustrations.